AF615050

STRUCTURE-ACTIVITY RELATIONSHIP ANALYSIS OF CHINESE ANTICANCER DRUGS AND RELATED PLANTS

by
Eric J. Lien and Wen Y. Li
Section of Biomedicinal Chemistry
School of Pharmacy
University of Southern California

Oriental Healing Arts Institute 1985
Long Beach, CA

STRUCTURE-ACTIVITY RELATIONSHIP ANALYSIS OF CHINESE ANTICANCER DRUGS AND RELATED PLANTS

ISBN: 0-941942-18-X
Printed in Taiwan, R.O.C.

Table of Contents

FOREWORD

Modern medicine began in 1858 when a German pathologist Rudolph Virchow (1828-1902) formulated the science of cellular pathology. Since then remarkable scientific advances in all areas have often been directly applied to medicine. Though today modern medicine has reached an advanced stage, it has, as yet, been unable to treat many illnesses effectively, most notably cancer.

Many scientists have employed advanced techniques to investigate the causes of cancer, but the results have not been so encouraging. In treating cancer, Western medicine adopts three basic methods: surgery, radiation therapy, and drug therapy. Drug therapy, the use of anticancer drugs, induces side effects in fifty to sixty-five percent of the cases, occasionally more. Regrettably, up to the present time no effective drug for cancer is known that does not adversely affect healthy cells. Despite many difficulties, the medical profession still hopes that an appropriate drug free from side effects will eventually be discovered.

Chinese medicine approaches cancer differently from Western medicine. Although Chinese medicine also employs "toxins to attack toxins", this method is by no means a major principle of treatment espoused in classic Chinese medical texts. In fact, Chinese medicine stresses an individual's "conformation", to which appropriate herbal formulas are prescribed. A conformation is a constellation of factors, including symptoms, signs, causes, nature and location of the illness, and the patient's physical condition. In brief, Chinese medicine aims to strengthen the body's ability to resist disease, and consequently when cancer invades the body, it naturally generates resistance. This point of view has been elaborated upon in my book *Treating Cancer with Chinese Herbs* (Oriental Healing Arts Institute, Los Angeles), in which various types of cancer and their therapeutic methods are discussed.

Professor Eric J. Lien has long been studying medicinal substances. His research interests range from natural products to physical organic chemistry to quantitative structure-activity relationships. As a specialist in chemical constituents and analysis of anticancer herbs, he has collected information, presented his research findings, and carefully reviewed and arranged these materials for our readers. Rich in content and different from any book on anticancer drugs, this book discusses in depth the relationships between anticancer Chinese drugs and their pharmacology, as its title implies. It further extols the efficacy of these drugs, thus taking the study of anticancer drugs a step further.

Professor Lien and Mrs. Lien were two of my outstanding students when I was teaching at National Taiwan University's School of Medicine from 1955-1965. He received his B.S. in Pharmacy in 1960 and his Ph.D. from the University of California at San Francisco in 1966. After completing post-doctoral training at Pomona College in 1968, he joined the faculty of the University of Southern California School of Pharmacy. He has written many articles for the Oriental Healing Arts Institute Bulletin and is currently a board member of OHAI.

Co-author Wen Y. Li, an associate of Professor Lien, graduated from Szechwen medical college in China. Li has published many articles on pharmaceutical preparations and analysis. In 1982 he came to the United States as a visiting scholar at the University of Southern California School of Pharmacy where he continues his research on quantitative structure-activity relationships and natural products.

We wish to express our gratitude to the authors for their kindness in granting the publication of their research papers which, we are sure, have made valuable contributions to the study of Chinese herbal medicine, particularly in the treatment of cancer.

We also wich to thank Wen Y. Li and Lin Ying for contributing the molecular structure diagrams, Paul Laurence and Jeannine E. Talley, Ph.D. for editing, Wang Shu-kuei for proofreading, and Lee Chung-jen for the cover design.

Hong-yen Hsu, Ph.D.
President
Oriental Healing Arts Institute

PREFACE

Traditional Chinese medicine depends mainly on empirical approaches. For centuries experimentation was done directly on patients without animal tests having been performed first. As a result, thousands of herbs, plants, and preparations have been handed down to contemporary practioners in China and many other parts of the world.

Only in the last few decades have the composition and efficacy of various Chinese herbs and plants been subjected to modern methods of analysis. In this book the authors have compiled those Chinese herbs and related plants having shown anticancer activity in established cell lines *in vitro* and/or animal models *in vivo*. Whenever possible clinical data are also included. Because of the vast amount of literature, it is not possible to include all data reported thus far. However, the authors have tried to include most representative groups of compounds from over 120 species of plants belonging to some 60 different families. The authors have also grouped many different Chinese drugs according to the general principles of bioorganic chemistry.

It is hoped that this work will stimulate further research in using traditional medicine or folk medicine as a clue to selection of species for research, and as an alternative to random and blind screening.

E. J. Lien
W. Y. Li
Los Angeles, 1984

1. Introduction

Natural products, especially compounds isolated from higher plants and microorganisms, have served as rich sources of novel drugs including anticancer drugs. In 1962 the National Cancer Institute in the United States (NCI) began a major effort to screen plant extracts. Table 1 shows the statistics on plant and animal extracts screened as of the end of 1980 by NCI.[1]

In China, some of the thousands of species of plants used either in traditional or Chinese folk herbal medicine have been screened. Many compounds with cytotoxic and/or antitumor activity have been discovered.[2-5] Although a few of them have been applied clinically or selected for further development as shown in Table 2, many compounds have so far shown good activity in the experimental models only.

To satisfy the continuing need for active compounds with novel structures and mechanisms of action, the quality of the screening methodology employed is a most important factor in analyzing a drug for any type of biological activity. Likewise, the structure-activity relationship analysis of these constituents is important for both rational use of Chinese medicine and for synthesis of novel drugs.

1.1 Screening methodology

Table 3 lists the tumor systems which have been used to

Table 1. Plant and Animal Extracts Screened by NCI Through December, 1980

Extract type	Samples screened	Confirmed active	Number of genera	Number of species
Plant	114,045	4,897 (4.3%)	1,551	3,394
Animal	16,196	660 (4.1%)	413	561

Table 2. Natural Products Analyzed or Used Clinically in China[4,5]

Vinca alkaloids: vinblastine (I), vincristine (II) and vindensine
Camptothecine (III) and 10-hydroxycamptothecine (IV)
Monocrotaline (V)
Indirubin (VI)
Harringtonine (VII)
Cantharidin (VIII) and N-hydroxycantharidinimide (a semisynthetic product) (IX)
Mixture of oridonin (X) and ponicidin (XI)
Diterpene-lactone mixture of *Tripterygium wilfordii* (XII)
Volatile oil of *Pelargonium geraveolens*[6]
Volatile oil of *Curcuma aromatica* (XIII)

screen the compounds discussed. Many of these tumor systems are no longer part of the current NCI screening program and have been dropped either because they are excessively sensitive and give a large number of false positive leads or because there is a poor correlation between the activity in the system and the known clinical efficacy.

The major bioassays currently in use in the NCI program are the KB and P-388 cell lines. The KB system measures toxicity to human cancer cells grown in cell cultures and has no necessary

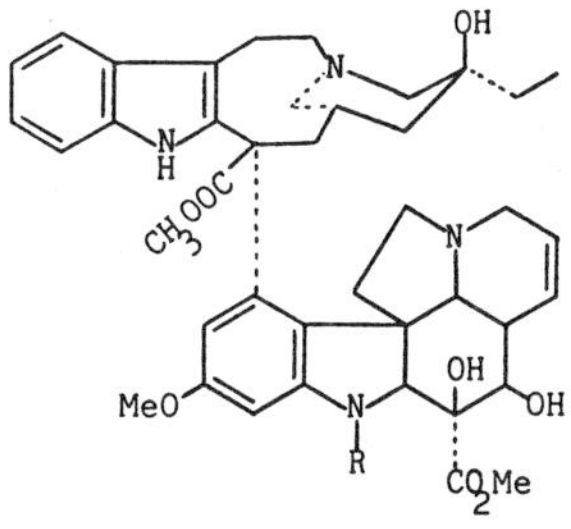

(I) R=CH_3 (II) R=CHO

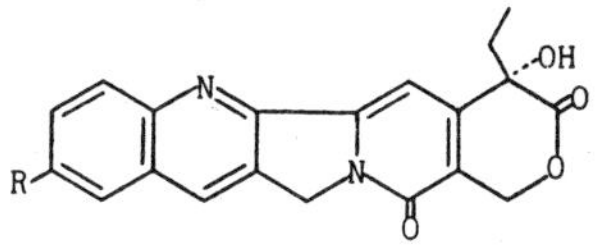

(III) R=H

(IV) R=OH

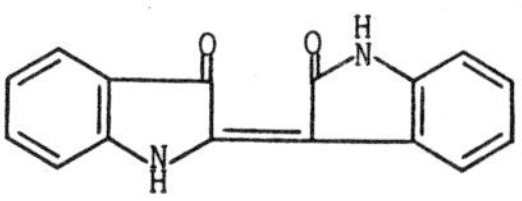

(VI)

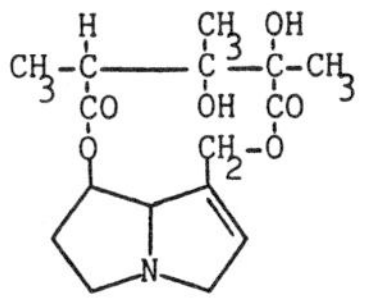

(V)

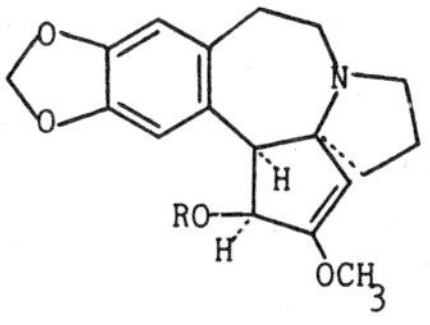

(VII) R=CH_3-C(OH)(CH_3)-$(CH_2)_2$-C(OH)(CO-)-CH_2-$COOCH_3$

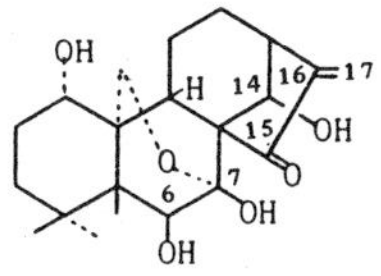

(X) 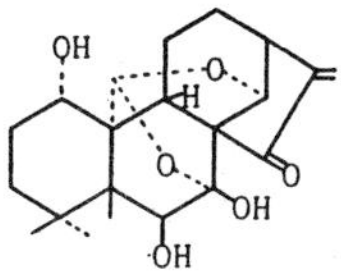 (XI) 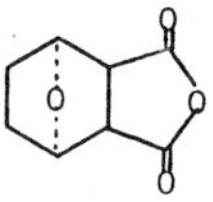 (VIII) 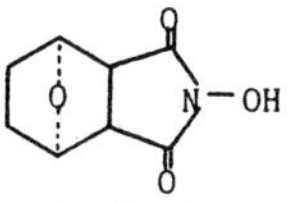 (IX)

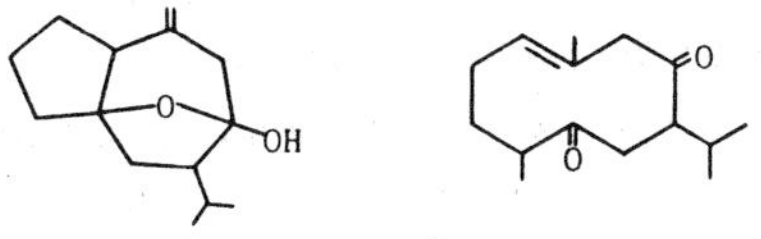

(XIII)

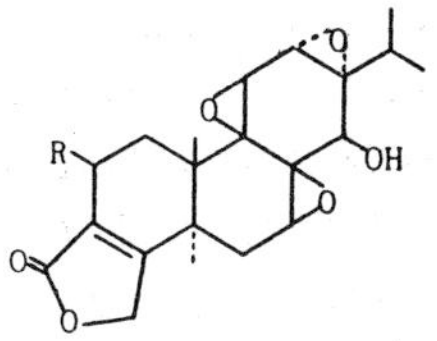

(XII) R=H; OH

Fig. 1 Chemical structures of natural products analyzed or used clinically in China

Table 3. NCI Tumor Systems

Tumor		Parameter measured	Minimal activity level (in T/C %)	Used in current screen
Code	Type			
B1	B16 melanosarcoma	survival	>125	yes
CA	Adenocarcinoma 755	tumor inhibition	<42	no
CD	CD8F1 mammary tumor	tumor inhibition	<42	yes
C6	Colon 26	survival	>140	yes
C8	Colon 38	tumor inhibition	<42	yes
DL	Dunning leukemia	survival	>125	no
EA	Ehrlich ascites	tumor inhibition	<42	no
KB	Carcinoma of naso-pharynx (cell culture)	cell growth inhibition	$ED_{50} < 4 \mu g/ml$	yes
LE	L-1210 lymphoid leukemia	survival	>125	yes
LL	Lewis lung carcinoma	survival (or inhibition)	>140 (or <42)	yes
P-4	P-1534 leukemia	survival	>125	no
PS	P-388 lymphocytic leukemia	survival	>120	yes
SA	Sarcoma-180	tumor inhibition	<42	no
WA	Walker carcino-sarcoma 256	tumor inhibition	<42	no

relationship to *in vivo* activity; KB activity alone is therefore not meaningful as a criterion for antitumor activity. However, within a series of compounds with *in vivo* activity, there is usually a fairly good correlation between the cytotoxicity of these compounds in the KB system and their *in vivo* activity, and the KB cells can be useful for analogues since the testing is rapid and requires only small amounts of materials.

It is also recognized that although the P-388 leukemia cells detect greater than 90% of known clinically effective agents, the

P-388 system is not perfect. Activity in P-388 leukemia has been deliberately chosen as the initial *in vivo* tumor system in the NCI current screen because it is quite sensitive and will pick up a large number of initially active compounds for more vigorous screening by other tumor systems. The P-388 system is therefore a prescreen detecting low-level activity and is not of much significance unless activity is also demonstrated in other systems.

The most dramatic development in screening in the last several years is the stem cell assay, which is now being developed as a screen for new compounds and as a validation test. This assay has proved to be closer to the human situation than any assay previously used in cancer drug screening, and currently the feeling is that it has a tremendous potential for detecting clinically effective agents.[1]

According to the NCI screening program, all novel compounds which are reproducibly active in the P-388 leukemia prescreen or which have been selected as bypass compounds should then go into tumor panel testing. The panel as presently constituted consists of eight systems, of which five are mouse tumor lines and three are human tumor lines carried in athymic mice.

Two activity levels for each tumor in the panel are determined for the active compounds as follows: a level of statistically significant activity (minimal activity) and a level of biologically important activity (Decision Network 2 level activity) as shown in Table 4. Activity levels are expressed as T/C percentage: the ratio of test group to control group animals.

Compounds meeting Decision Network 2 level activity in the panel become candidates for clinical trials.

Table 5 shows the status of plant-derived compounds currently in clinical trials or those which have passed Decision Network 2 activity or are candidates for advanced preclinical development.

Table 4. NCI Tumor Panel Systems and Activity Criteria (ILS = Increase in Lifespan, TWI = Tumor Weight Inhibition)

Tumor		Evaluation parameter	Activity level in (T/C %)	
Code	Type		Minimal	DN2
B16	B16 melanocarcinoma	ILS	125	150
CD	CD8F1 mammary	TWI	20	0
C8	Colon 38	TWI	⩽42	⩽10
LE	L1210 lymphoid leukemia	ILS	125	150
LL	Lewis lung carcinoma	ILS	140	150
C2	CX-1 colon xenograft	TWI	⩽20	⩽10
LK	LX-1 lung xenograft	TWI	⩽20	⩽10
MB	MX-1 breast xenograft	TWI	⩽20	⩽10

Table 5. Drugs in Advanced Development[1]

Drug	Status	Results
Maytansine	Phase II trials	Little activity
Bruceantin	Phase II trials	Minimal activity
Indicine-N-oxide	Phase II trials ongoing	Good responses in leukemia
Homoharringtonine	Phase I trials	
Taxol	Toxicology studies	
Ellipticine	Oral toxicology studies	
4-β-hydroxy-withanolide E	Formulation development	

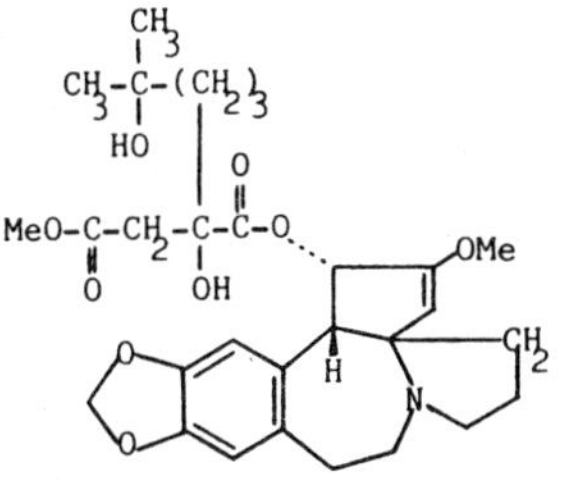

Homoharringtonine

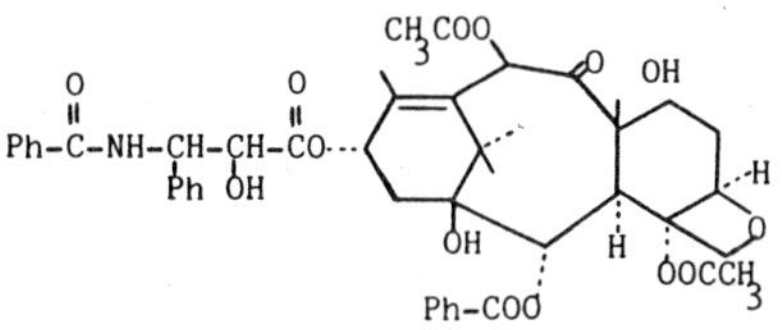

Taxol

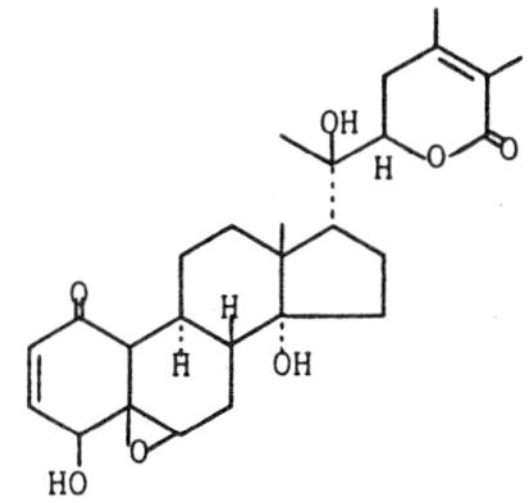

4-β-hydroxy-withanolide E

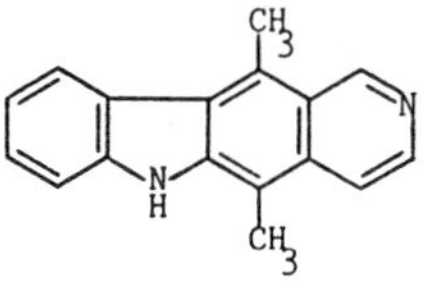

Ellipticine

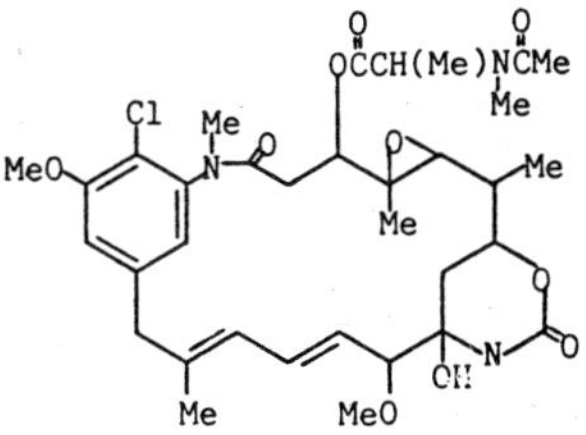

Maytansine

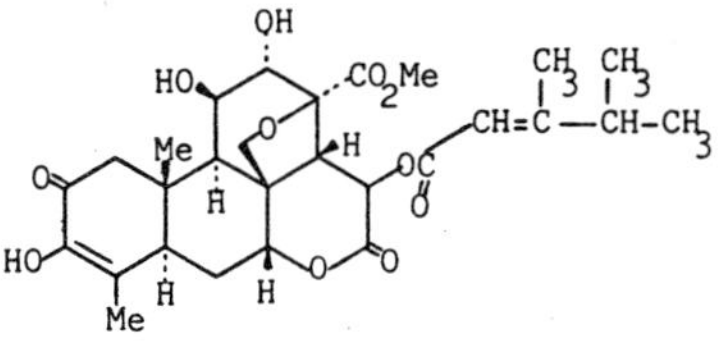

Bruceantin

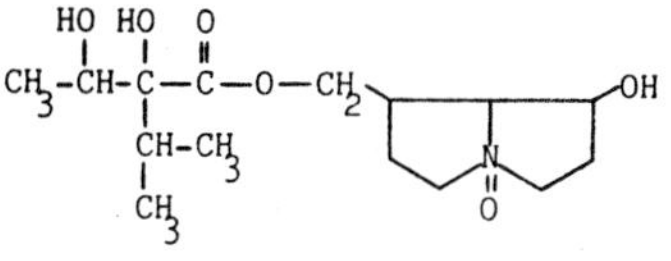

Indicine, N-oxide

Fig. 2 Molecular structures of drugs in advanced development

1.2 Structure-activity relationship analysis

Natural compounds with cytotoxic and/or antitumor activity belong to various categories based on their chemical structures. The most commonly found active principles are terpenes and alkaloids, in which the presence of certain common structural features or functional groups responsible for their activity can be found in many cases. The mechanisms of action of some anticancer drugs including those occurring in plants are shown in Figure 3.

This book presents a survey of the active constituents of Chinese herbs with anticancer activity and their structure-activity relationships (SAR). Over 120 species of plants belonging to some 60 different families are used either in Chinese traditional or folk medicine to treat cancer.

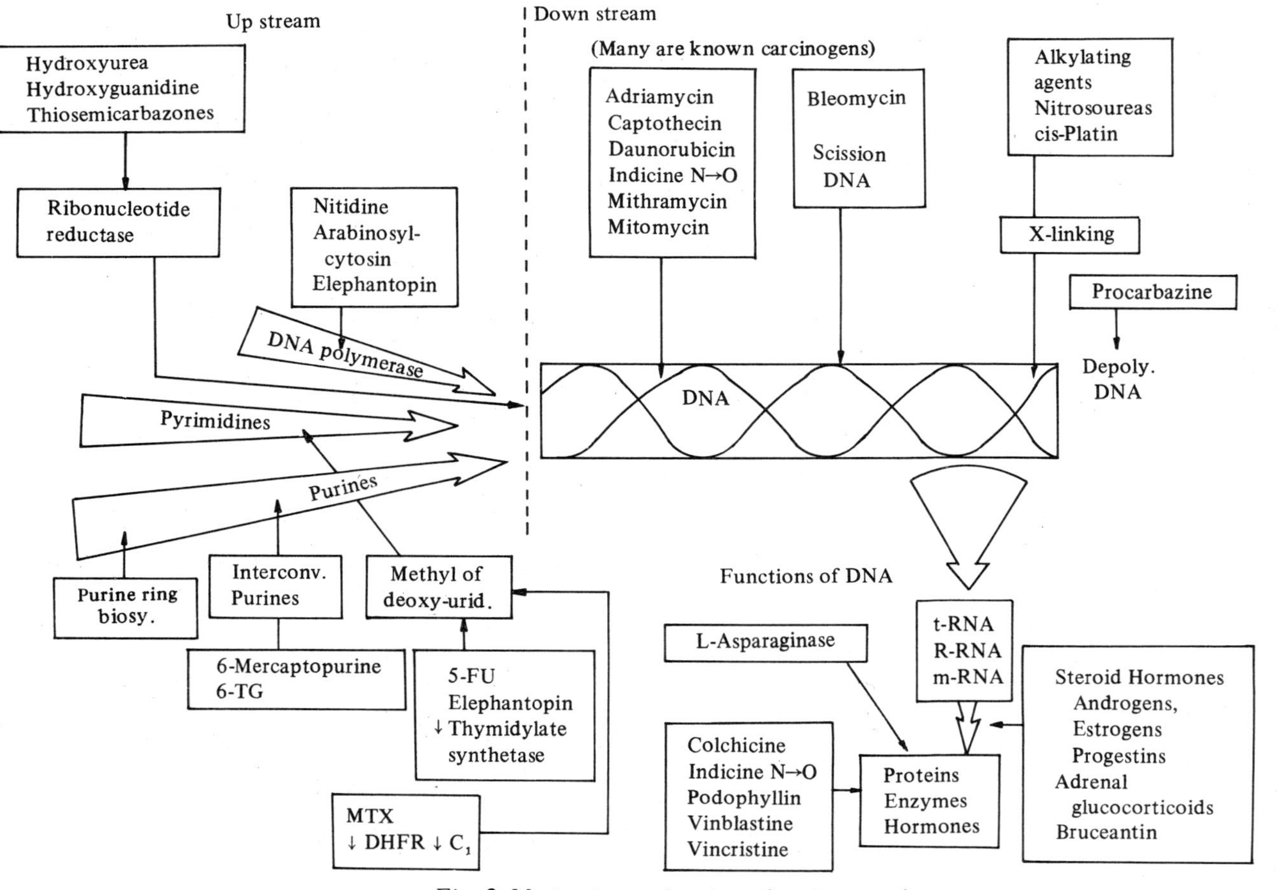

Fig. 3 Mechanisms of action of anticancer drugs

2. Sesquiterpene

A large number of sesquiterpenes, mainly derived from plants in the families of Compositae (90%) and Magnoliaceae (10%), have been evaluated as cytotoxic. Some of them exhibit activity *in vivo* against P-388 leukemia and other tumor systems. All of these compounds are derived biosynthetically from trans-fornesyl pyrophosphate (t-FPP) and can be classified structurally into five major groups based on their carbon skeleton as shown in Figure 4.

As shown in Table 6 through 10, these compounds generally contain one or more active groups which can be attacked by a biological nucleophilic macromolecule, resulting in alkylation of the essential biomolecules. The most common active group is the α-methylene-γ-lactone.

It has been found[9] that a number of sesquiterpene lactones containing the α-methylene-γ-lactone moiety are potent inhibitors of Walker-256 carcinosarcoma and Ehrlich ascites tumor growth and marginal inhibitors of P-388 lymphocytic leukemia and Lewis lung tumor growth. Comparison of the relative cytotoxicities of these sesquiterpene lactones and their derivatives has demonstrated that the electrophilic α-methylene-γ-lactone function is essential for maximum activity. *In vitro* aerobic basal respiration and oxidative phosphorylation processes of Ehrlich ascites were inhibited by these agents. The enzymes, deoxyribonucleic acid, polymerase, and thymidylate synthetase were also inhibited. The tumor inhibitory α-methylene-γ-lactones were also shown to inhibit phosphofructokinase and glycogen synthetase. Research has

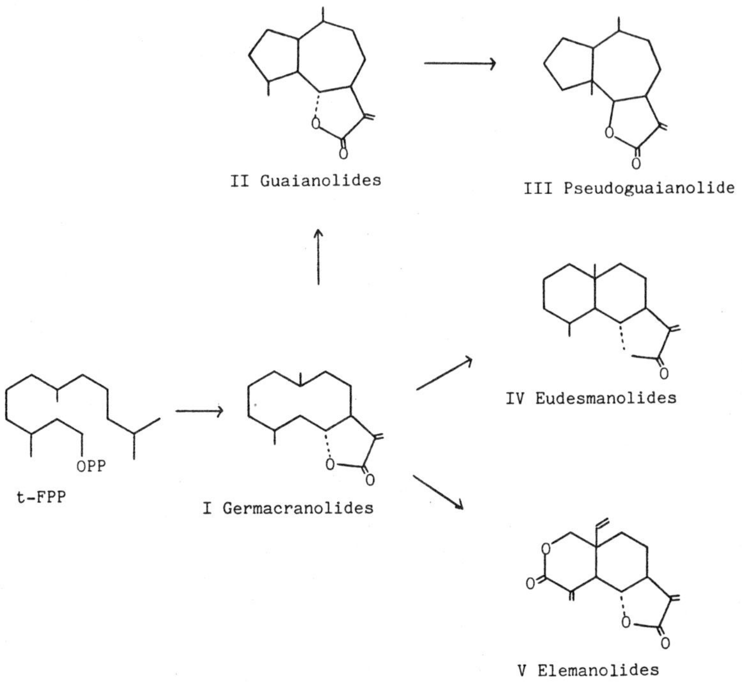

II Guaianolides

III Pseudoguaianolide

IV Eudesmanolides

t-FPP

OPP

I Germacranolides

V Elemanolides

Fig. 4 The carbon skeletons of the five major groups of sesquiterpenes derived from biosynthesis of trans-fornesyl pyrophosphate.

confirmed that the inhibition of these biochemical parameters results from their reaction with the essential SH groups of these enzymes[10-13] (Figure 5).

However, a majority of the hundreds of sesquiterpene lactones proved to be cytotoxic and antileukemic only *in vitro;* a single reactive group such as the α-methylene-γ-lactone function is not sufficient to impart significant *in vivo* activity.

The rate constants for reaction of α-methylene-γ-lactones with cysteine at pH 7.4 range from about 100 LM^{-1} min^{-1} to 15,000 LM^{-1} min.$^{-1}$ This large difference in rates was chiefly attributed to neighboring group effects. Generally, α-methylene-γ-lactone containing an adjacent -OH or -OCOR group had a rate of reaction more than 720 LM^{-1} min,$^{-1}$ while the natural products with significant *in vivo* activity showed a rate of reaction greater than 1,000 LM^{-1} min.$^{-1}$ For example, elephantopin and related

2.1 Germacranolides

Table 6. Cytotoxicity and Antitumor Activity of Germacranolides

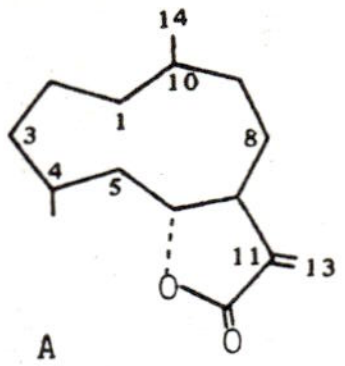

	Compound		Structure	KB ED_{50} (μg/ml)	*In vivo* T/C% (mg/kg)	Source
1.	Costunolide	[A]	$\Delta^{1,10}; \Delta^{4,5}$	0.69		*Saussurea lappa*
2.	Eupatolide	[A]	$\Delta^{1,10}; \Delta^{4,5}$; 8-β-OH	0.5-1.3	L-1210 160	*Eupatorium cannabinum*
3.	Lipiferolide	[A]	$\Delta^{1,10}$; 4,5-β-epoxy; 8-β-$OCOCH_3$	0.16		*Liriodendron tulipifera*
4.	Liatrin	[A]	$\Delta^{1,2}; \Delta^{4,5}$; 3, 10-epoxy; 3-α-OH; 8-β-$OOC(CH_2OAc)CHCH_3$	1.62	PS 175	*Liatris chapmanii*
5.	Tamaulipin A	[A]	$\Delta^{1,10}; \Delta^{4,5}$; 2-α-OH	1.26		*Ambrosia canfertiflora*
6.	Tamaulipin B	[A]	$\Delta^{1,10}; \Delta^{4,5}$; 3-β-OH	2.60		
7.	Peroxycostunolide	[A]	$\Delta^{4,5}; \Delta^{10,14}$; 1-β-OOH	2.70	WA 50	
8.	Hydroxycostunolide	[A]	$\Delta^{4,5}; \Delta^{10,14}$; 1-β-OH	2.80	PS 160 (10)	
9.	Elephantopin	[B]	$\Delta^{1,10}; \Delta^{11,13}$; 8-β-$OOCC(Me)CH_2$	0.3	WA 12	*Elephantopus elatus*
10.	Elephantin	[B]	$\Delta^{1,10}; \Delta^{11,13}$; 8-α-$OCOCHC(Me)_2$	0.94		
11.	Tetrahydroelephantopin	[B]	$\Delta^{1,10}$; 8-α-$OCOCH(Me)_2$	72		
12.	Hexahydroelephantopin	[B]	8-α-$OCOCH(Me)_2$	<100		

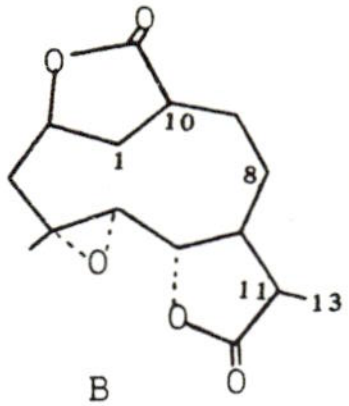

2.2 Guianolides

Table 7. Cytotoxicity of guianolides

A

B

	Compound		Structure	*In vitro* (μg/ml)	ED_{50}	Source
13.	Arteglasin-A	[A]	$\Delta^{1,10}$; 3β, 4β-epoxy; 8-β-$OCOCH_3$	HEP-2*	1.92	*Artemisia douglasiana*
14.	Euparotin	[A]	$\Delta^{3,4}$; 2-β-OH; 5-α-OH; 10, 14-epoxy; 8-β-OCOC(Me)$CHCH_3$	KB	0.21	*Eupatorium rotundifolium*
15.	Gaillardin	[B]	$\Delta^{8,10}$; 4-α-OH; 2-α-OAc	KB	2.3	*Gaillardia pulchella*
16.	Xerantholide	[B]	$\Delta^{4,5}$; 3 = O	KB	1.5	*Xeranthenum cylindraceum*

*Human epidermal carcinoma of the larynx.

2.3 Pseudoguaianolides

Table 8. Cytotoxicity and Antitumor Activity of Pseudoguaianalides

A. B

	Compound		Structure	KB ED_{50} (μg/ml)	PS T/C (mg/kg)	Source
17.	Ambrosin	[A]	$\Delta^{2,3}$; 4 = O	0.04	180 (35)	*Ambrosia maritinia*
18.	Multigilin	[B]	$\Delta^{2,3}$; 4=O; 9-β-OH; 6-α-OCOC(Me)=CH(Me)		160 (12.5)	*Baileya multiradiata*
19.	Helenalin	[B]	$\Delta^{2,3}$; 4 = O; 6-α-OH	0.19	127 (25) WA 316 LL 142	*Helenium autumnale*
20.	Gaillardilin	[B]	2-β-OH; 6-β-OAc; 3β, 4β-epoxy	2.2		*Gaillardia pinnatifida*
21.	Mexicanin-I	[B]	$\Delta^{2,3}$; 4 = O; 6-β-OH	0.33; 1.90		
22.	Aromaticin	[B]	$\Delta^{2,3}$; 4 = O	0.34; 2.0		

2.4 Eudesmanolides

Table 9. Cytotoxicity of Eudesmanolides

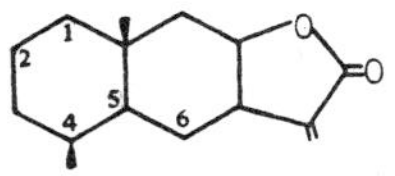

A

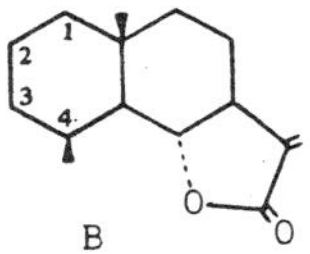

B

	Compound		Structure	KB ED_{50} (μg/ml)	Source
23.	Alantolactone	[A]	$\Delta^{5,6}$	1.4	*Inula helenium*
24.	Ivalin	[A]	$\Delta^{4,5}$; 2-α-OH	0.7	*Iva macrocephala*
25.	Santamarin	[B]	$\Delta^{3,4}$; 1-β-OH	1.1	*Michelia compressa*

2.5 Elemanolides

Table 10. Cytotoxicity and Antitumor Activity of Elemanolides

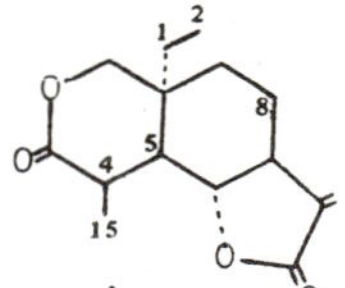

	Compounds		Structure	KB ED_{50} (μg/ml)	*In vivo* T/C (mg/kg)	Source
26.	Vernolepin	[A]	$\Delta^{1,2}$; $\Delta^{4,15}$; 8-α-OH	2.0	WA 68 (12)	*Vernonia hymenolepsis*
27.	Vernolepin methacrylate	[A]	$\Delta^{1,2}$; $\Delta^{4,15}$; 8-α-OCOC(Me)=CH_2	0.42		
28.	Vernolepin acetate	[A]	$\Delta^{1,2}$; $\Delta^{4,15}$; 8-α-OAc	2.70		
29.	Dihydrovernolepin	[A]	$\Delta^{4,15}$; 8-α-OH	2.00		
30.	Vernomenin	[B]	$\Delta^{1,2}$; $\Delta^{4,5}$; 6-α-OH	35.0	37 (8)	*Vernonia guineensia*

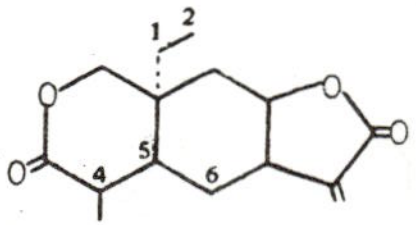

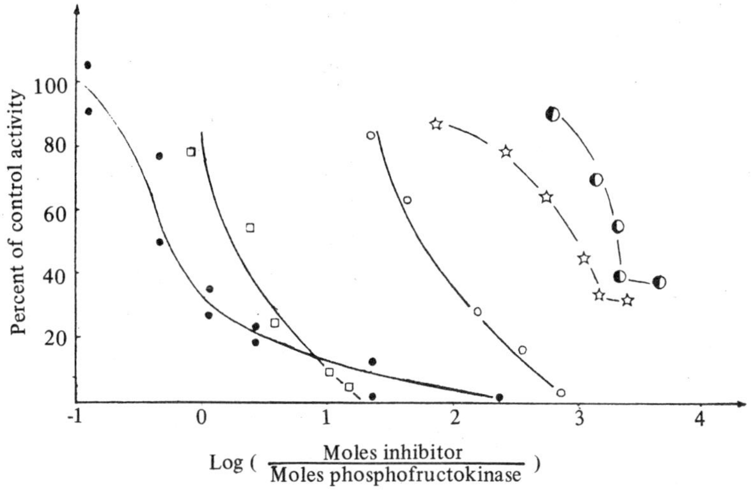

Fig. 5 Inhibition of phosphofructokinase by tumor inhibitors and by sulfhydryl reagent – Ellman's reagent [5,5′-dithiobis-(2-nitrobenzoic acid)] From reference 13.

- ● Ellman's reagent
- □ Taxodione
- ○ Taxodone
- ☆ Euparotin acetate
- ◐ Vernolepin

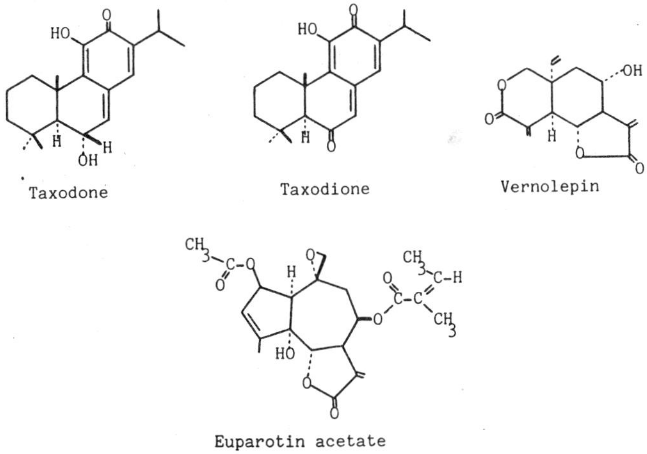

Taxodone

Taxodione

Vernolepin

Euparotin acetate

Fig. 6 Chemical structures of taxodone, taxodione, vernolepin, and euparotin acetate

compounds are known to exist in *Elephantopus elatus, E. scaber* (丁茄杇 , *ding-chai-wu*) and *E. mollis* (地膽草 , *ti-tan-t'sao*) of the Compositae. Among these, elephantopin (KB ED_{50} = 0.3 μg/ml, T/C = 171% at 40 mg/kg against P-388) has been selected for further tumor panel evaluation by NCl.[11] Molephantinin was also shown to be active against Walker-256 carcinosarcoma growth in rats at 2.5 mg/kg/day resulting in a T/C of 397%. The agent was also active against P-388 lymphocytic leukemia and Ehrlich ascites growth.[12] This may be due to combination of α-methylene-γ-lactone function with an epoxide and α,β-unsaturated ester. The rate constants for the addition of cysteine to elephantopin is 2,600 LM^{-1} min^{-1}.

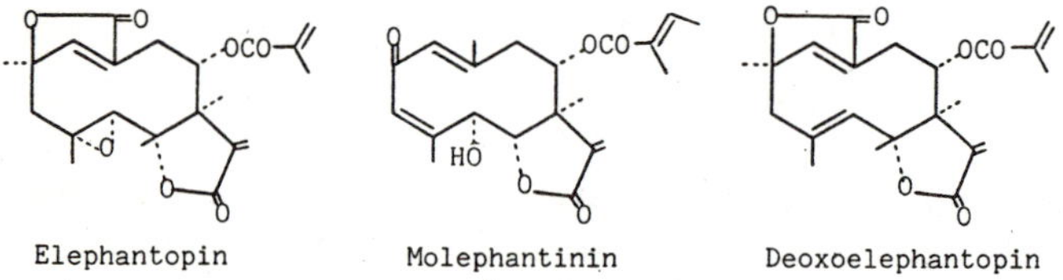

Elephantopin Molephantinin Deoxoelephantopin

Fig. 7 Chemical structures of elephantopin, molephantinin, and deoxoelephantopin

This type of compound containing the allylic ester side chain was demonstrated to have higher activity, perhaps due to enhanced membrane transport of these compounds. The unsaturated ester moiety might also act as an alkylating function, as shown in the Michael addition between elephantopin and cysteine.[13]

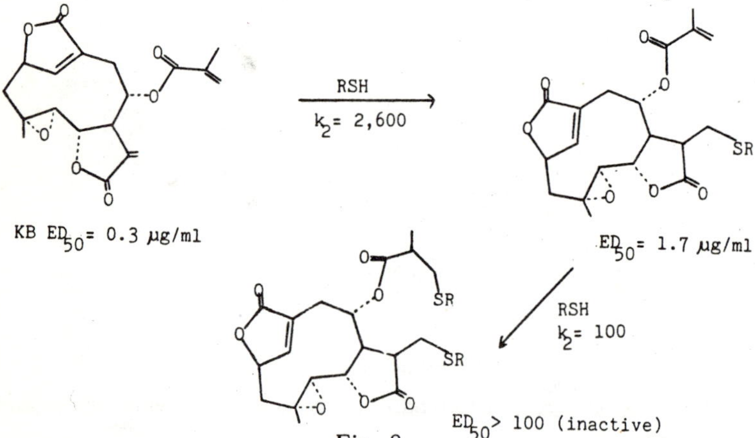

RSH k_2 = 2,600

KB ED_{50} = 0.3 μg/ml

ED_{50} = 1.7 μg/ml

RSH k_2 = 100

ED_{50} > 100 (inactive)

Fig. 8

When a lactone moiety lacking an adjacent -OH group or the ester chain was saturated, its activity was consistently less; replacement of one hydrogen on the α-methylene group by alkyl, alkylamino, alkoxy group resulted in a decrease in reactivity with cysteine, and loss of cytotoxic activity.

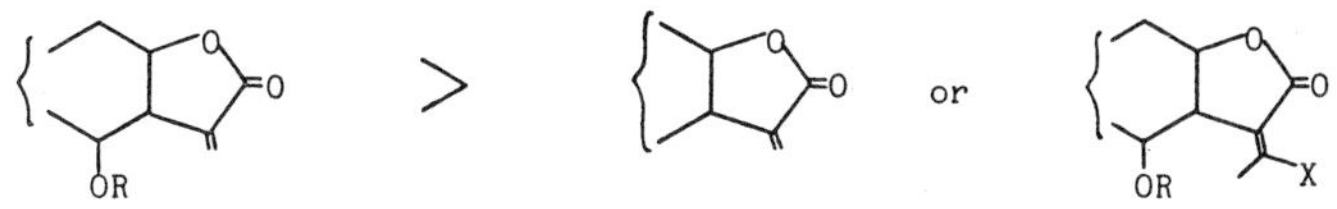

R=H or Acyl > (or) X=Alkyl, Alkylamino or Alkoxy

Fig. 9

In addition to α-methylene-γ-lactone moiety, the α,β-unsaturated cyclopentenone ring, α-epoxycyclopentanone, and α-methylene cyclopentanone systems are the essential functional groups for inhibition of these biochemical parameters mentioned above:

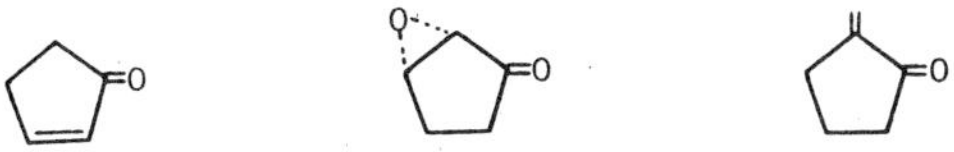

Fig. 10

The most significantly active compounds are multifunctional, and placement of the hydroxyl group at certain positions on the ring appears to substantially increase both T/C and potency, for example:

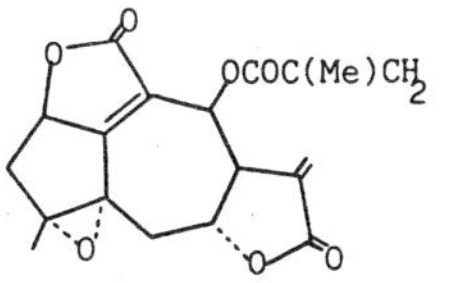

Elephantopine

Ps: T/C = 160% (10 mg/kg)
171% (40 mg/kg)

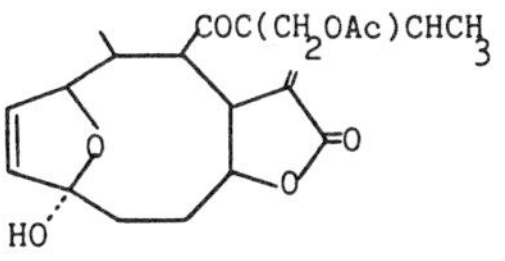

Liatrin

Ps : T/C = 157% (8 mg/kg)

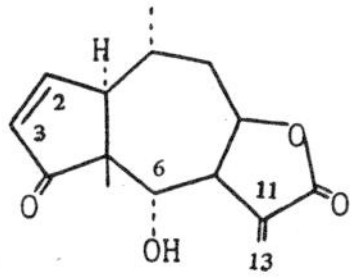

Helenalin

Ps: T/C = 168% (8 mg/kg)
200% (3 mg/kg)

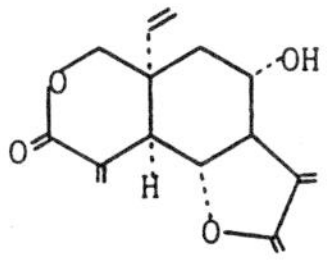

Vernolepin

Ps: T/C = 145% (1.88 mg/kg)

Fig. 11

Helenolides containing both α-methylene-γ-lactone moiety and α, β-unsaturated cyclopentenone ring have high antitumor activity.[14-16]

Table 11. Cytotoxicity of Helenolides Against Human Epidermoid Carcinoma of the Larynx (Hep-2)

Compounds	Hep-2 ED_{50} (μg/ml)
Helenalin	0.10
2,3-dihydrohelenalin	3.84
11,13-dihydrohelenalin	0.80
2,3,11,13-tetrahydrohelenalin	>40.0
2,3-epoxyhelenalin	0.11
1,2-epoxyhelenalin	0.53
1,2,11,13-diepoxyhelenalin	0.50

Helenalin isolated from *Helenium autumnale* (堆心菊 , *tuei-hsin-zhu*) is the most active component of this group. It exhibited significant antitumor activity against WM-256 ascites carcinoma (T/C = 316% at 2.5 mg/kg/day), P-388 (T/C = 127% at 25 mg/kg/day), and Lewis lung cancer (T/C = 142% at 25 mg/kg/day).

From the findings shown in table 11, structural-activity relationship studies have indicated the following: (1) The α,β-unsaturated cyclopentenone ring and α-methylene-γ-lactone system all contributed significantly to the *in vitro* and *in vivo* activities, but the former was more important. Hydrogenation of $\Delta^{2,3}$ resulted in a profound diminution of antitumor activity. (2) The cytotoxicity of helenalin only showed slight diminution when the double bond – either $\Delta^{2,3}$ or $\Delta^{11,13}$ – was reverted into an epoxyl group, indicating the epoxyl group is also an active center. (3) The esterification of a 6-α-OH group of helenalin, especially the one bearing a conjugated ester group, will increase significantly its cytotoxicity.

In addition, some non-lactone sesquiterpene derivatives have also been shown to be active in some antitumor test systems. For example, curcumol and curdione isolated from the volatile oil of Chinese plant *Curcuma aromatica* (莪朮 , *e-zhu*) (Zingiberaceae) have shown an inhibitory effect on sarcoma 180 in mice. This drug has been used to treat the early stage of cervical cancer.[11]

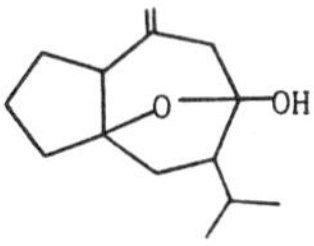

Curcumol

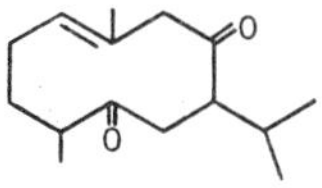

Curdione

Fig. 12

The chinese drug *Atractylodes macrocephala* (白朮 , *bei-zhu*) (Compositae) showed activity against esophageal cancer (Ca 109) *in vitro*. The principles were identified as atractylon and butenolide B, among others.[11]

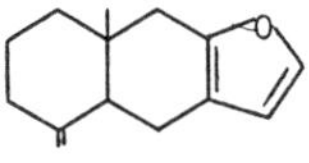

Atractylon

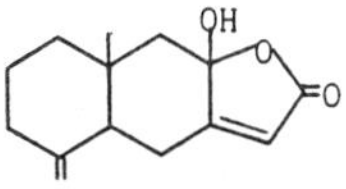

Butenolide B

Fig. 13

3. Diterpenes

3.1 Quassinoids (See Figure 14)

The bitter principles isolated from many genera of the Simaroubaceae family have shown a high degree of antileukemia activity in animals.[17-19] For example, the series of bruceolides, isolated from *Brucea* species, has been proven to have significant inhibitory activity against several experimental neoplasms, including cells derived from the human carcinoma of the nasopharynx (KB), Walker-256 intramuscular carcinoma in the rat, and P-388 lymphocytic leukemia in the mouse (PS).

Attention has focused on the quassinoids in recent years because several of them have shown promise as anticancer agents. In particular, bruceantin, one quassinoid isolated from *B. antidysenterica,* has been placed on phase II clinical trials by the U.S. National Cancer Institute.[11]

The Chinese drug (鴉膽子 , *ya-tan-tzu*) is the seed of *B. javanica* (L.) Merr. All parts of the plant are bitter, especially the seed and root.

Two glycosidic bruceolides (bruceosides-A and -B) and five bruceolide derivatives (brusatol, bruceine-D and -E, dehydrobruceine-B, and brucea-ketolic acid) have been isolated from *B. javanica* fruits.[20-23] These bruceolide derivatives together with bruceines-A, -B, -C, -F, and -G were previously reported to be contained in material identified as *B. amarissima.*[21] In addition, it has been reported that the potent antineoplastic bruceolides, bruceantin, and bruceantinol, previously only isolated from *B. antidysenterica* and *B. quineasia,* have also been isolated together

Fig. 14 Basic structure of quassinoids

with bruceantarin, dehydrobruceine-A, and dihydrobruceine-A from *B. javanica,* a species introduced into Fiji.[21]

Tests have shows that bruceoside-A and -B possess significant antileukemic activity (T/C ⩾ 120%) in P-388 lymphocytic leukemia (T/C = 156 and 132%), at the 6 and 1.5 mg/kg/day levels, respectively.[24]

Among these bruceolides, bruceantin and bruceantinol are potent antileukemic compounds and have shown significant antineoplastic activity against a series of test neoplasms. Bruceantin possesses high activity against P-388 lymphocytic leukemia in the mouse with a T/C value consistently greater than 200, and with cytotoxicity usually observed at a concentration of 10^{-2} μg/ml. It also showed significant inhibitory activity against the L-1210 lymphoid leukemia and against two solid murine tumor systems: the Lewis lung carcinoma and the B-16 melanocarcinoma.[11,17,25,26] Brusatol, bruceine-B and -D also significantly inhibit P-388 lymphocytic leukemic cell DNA and protein synthesis in cell culture. Bruceine-A is highly toxic to TLX-5 mice lymphoma cells, and bruceine-D inhibits the growth of Walker-256 carcinosarcoma in rats with a T/C = 144% at the 0.5 mg/kg/day level. It and bruceine-E showed antimalarial action too. In comparison with bruceantin, they demonstrated lower activity in the same system (Table 12), possibly due to a lower lipophilicity in the side chain which may be a requirement for transport across cell membranes.

The antileukemic activity of the bruceolides varies greatly with the nature of the C-15 ester substituent. Bruceantin and bruceantinol which bear an α, β-unsaturated ester group showed potent antileukemic activity, bruceantarin with a benzoate ester, and dihydrobruceantin with a saturated aliphatic ester moiety

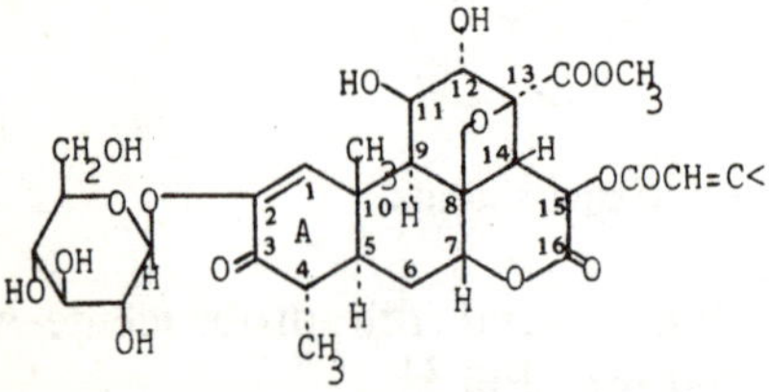

Bruceoside-A

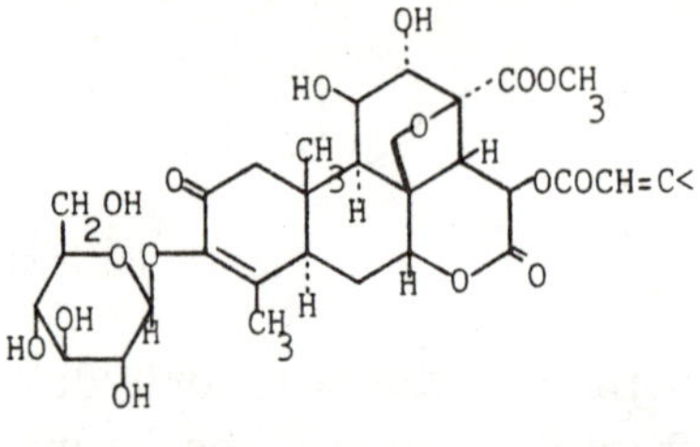

Bruceoside-B

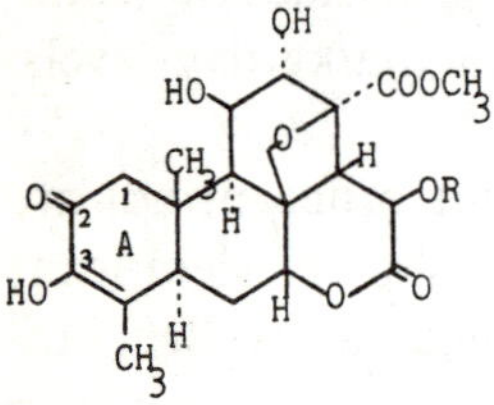

Bruceolide	R=H
Bruceine A	$R=COCH_2CH(CH_3)_2$
Bruceine B	$R=COCH_3$
Bruceine C	$R=COCH_2-CH(CH_3)-C(OH)(CH_3)_2$
Bruceantin	$R=COCH=C(CH_3)CH(CH_3)_2$
Bruceantinol	$R=COCH=C(CH_3)C(OH)(CH_3)_2$
Bruceantarin	$R=COC_6H_5$
Brusatol	$R=COCH=C(CH_3)_2$

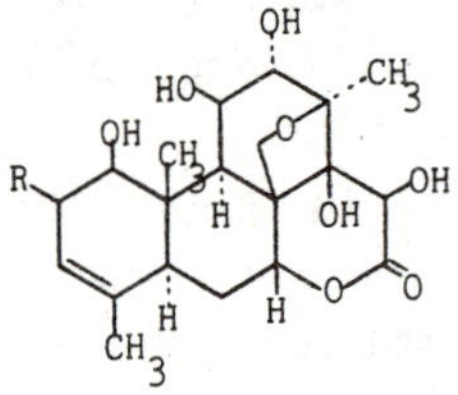

Bruceine D R= =O

Bruceine E R= α-OH

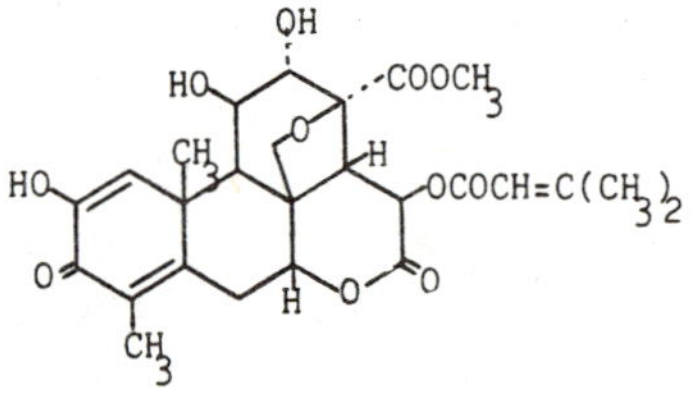

Dehydrobruceine A
$R=COCH_2CH(CH_3)_2$

Dehydrobruceine B
$R=COCH_3$

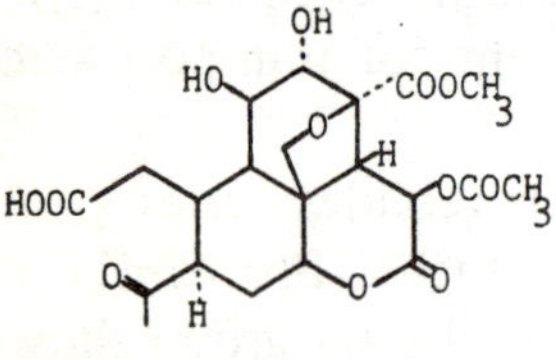

Bruceaketolic acid

Fig. 15

Table 12. Activities Against P-388 Lymphocytic Leukemia of Bruceolide Derivatives

Compound	Doses (mg/kg/day)	T/C % (in mouse)
Bruceoside-A and -B	1.5 6.0	132 156
Brusatol	0.125 0.5 1.0 2.0	158 161 198 191
Bruceine-C	1.0	152
Bruceantin	0.5 2.0	197 225
Bruceantinol	0.25 2.0	200 238
Bisbrusatolyl succinate	0.6	217
Bisbrusatolyl malonate	0.3 0.6 1.0	215 272 213
6-Senecioyloxychaparrinone	1.0	198
Holacanthone	0.13	227
Glaucarubinone	0.50	231

showed moderated activity, while bruceine-B with the smaller acetate ester and bruceolide with no ester at all showed only marginal antileukemic activity. The C-15 ester moiety probably serves as a carrier group in processes such as membrane transport of the drug into intact cells or complex formation.[17]

Bruceoside-A and -B are two quassinoid glucosides which have been demonstrated to have antileukemic activities. They can be extracted by methanol in good yield from the seeds of *Brucea javanica* defatted by n-hexane. Acid hydrolysis of both bruceoside-A and -B with 3N sulfuric acid-methanol (1:1) yielded D-glucose and brusatol as the aglycon. The structure and stereochemistry of brusatol are identical to those of bruceantin except for the slight difference in the C-15 ester side chain.

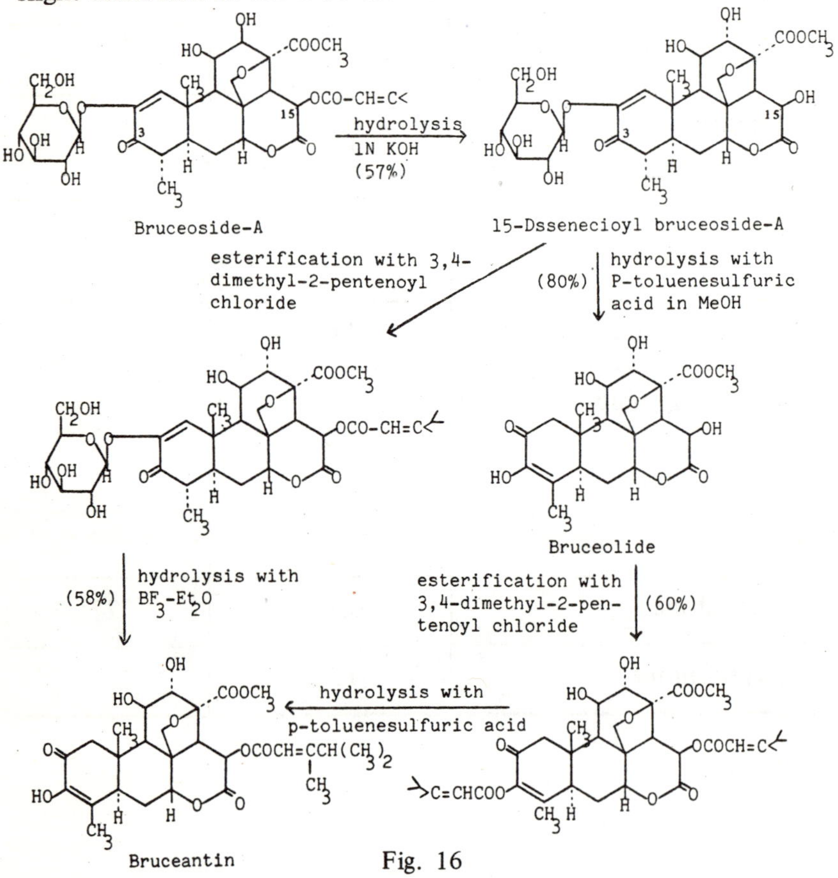

Bruceoside-A → hydrolysis 1N KOH (57%) → 15-Dssenecioyl bruceoside-A

15-Dssenecioyl bruceoside-A → esterification with 3,4-dimethyl-2-pentenoyl chloride

15-Dssenecioyl bruceoside-A → (80%) hydrolysis with P-toluenesulfuric acid in MeOH → Bruceolide

→ (58%) hydrolysis with BF_3-Et_2O → Bruceantin

Bruceolide → esterification with 3,4-dimethyl-2-pentenoyl chloride (60%) → hydrolysis with p-toluenesulfuric acid → Bruceantin

Fig. 16

In view of the importance of 3,4-dimethyl-2-pentenoyl ester moiety for the antileukemic activity of bruceantin, bruceoside-A has been converted by two methods to bruceantin as shown in Figure 16, based upon selective esterification and hydrolysis at C-3 and C-15 hydroxyl groups.[27]

In addition to the importance of the ester groups at either C-15 or C-6, it was concluded that the Δ^3-2-oxo moiety in ring A, the methylenoxy bridge and the hydroxyl moieties at either C_1 or C_3 and C_{12} are required for antileukemic activity of quassinoids. These include compounds isolated from other genera of the family Simaroubaceae, such as 6α-senecioyloxychaparrinone, holacanthone, glancarublone, and related compounds other than bruceolides.[12,28]

The importance of the Michael-type addition of model biological nucleophiles (selected enzyme sulfydrol groups) to highly electrophilic conjugated systems, such as α-methylene-γ-lactones,[29] α-methylene-cyclopentanone,[30] α, β-unsaturated-γ-lactones, and epoxide-function with a neighboring -OH group[31]

Table 13. The Sources and Structures of Holacanthone and Related Compounds

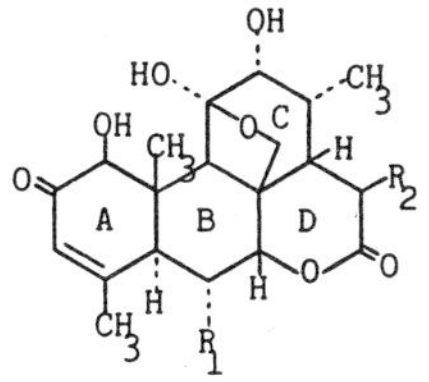

Compound	Structure	Source
6α-senecioyloxy-chaparrinone	R_1=-OCO-=< R_2=H	*Simaba multiflora*
Holacanthone	R_1=H R_2=OAc	*Holacanthus emoryii*
Glancarubinone	R_1=H R_2=O_2C-C(OH)(CH_3)-Et	*Simarouba glauca*

in relation to the cytotoxicity of several classes of terpenoides, has been demonstrated. The unsaturated ketone group undoubtedly acts as an alkylating agent.[32] Thus, saturation of the conjugated Δ^3-double bond or reduction of the ketone group in the quassinoids is accompanied by a profound lessening in cytotoxicity of the resulting dihydroquassinoid derivatives. In contrast, the neighboring hydroxyl group at C_1 or C_3 may enhance the reactivity of the conjugated ketone toward biological nucleophiles through intramolecular hydrogen bonding as shown below:[34]

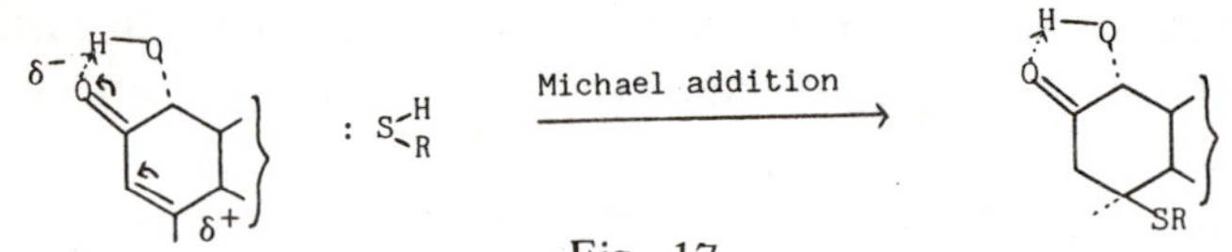

Michael addition

Fig. 17

In view of the requirements of the functional alkylating enone O=C–C=CH– system and the ester moiety for enhanced antileukemic activity of bruceantin, a minor modification by combining two intact active quassinoids via a diester linkage may yield highly active antileukemic agents with reduced toxicity, thus the corresponding bisbrusatol and bisbruceantin esters with bifunctional groups have been synthesized by treatment with malonyl dichloride and succinyl dichloride.[24]

Of the semisynthetic compounds, the bisbrusatolyl esters were in general more potent than brusatol, especially the succinate and malonate with a T/C of 217 and 272, respectively. The C-3 esters of brusatol and bruceantin were also found to be as active or more active than brusatol or bruceantin in general, but esterification of the C-11 and C-12 hydroxyl groups resulted in marked reduction of activity.[24]

It has been shown that the primary mode of action of bruceolides is through inhibition of protein synthesis. At a concentration of 5×10^{-9} M, bruceantin inhibits protein synthesis in HeLa cells by 90% and inhibits DNA synthesis by 40%, but shows little effect on RNA synthesis. This inhibitory action is not reversible in cell cultures.[35-37]

A series of brusatol, bisbrusatol, and bruceantin esters was also shown to inhibit DNA and protein synthesis in P-388 lym-

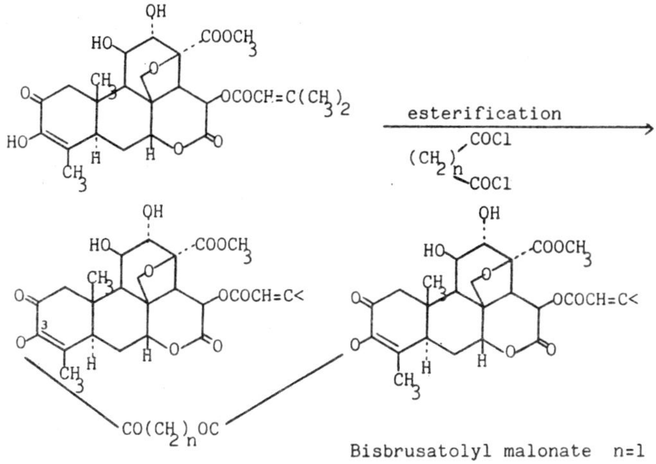

Bisbrusatolyl malonate n=1

Bisbrusatolyl succinate n=2

Fig. 18

phocytic leukemia cells, and the ability was correlated with their antineoplastic activity. Compounds which produced high T/C values successfully suppressed a number of enzymes involved in nucleic acid metabolism, for example, DNA polymerase and dihydrofolate reductase, suggesting that quassinoids are elongation inhibitors of tumor cells, and that the free 80S ribosome is the site of binding by quassinoid.[38,39]

Preclinical toxicological studies of bruceantin performed in dogs and monkeys disclosed significant acute gastrointestinal toxicity manifesting as anorexia, emesis, enteritis, and hepatocellular damage. In addition, it was found to cause hematuria, bradycardia, cardiac arrhythmia, hypothermia, and ataxia. Phase I clinical studies of bruceantin have shown that gastrointestinal toxicity was commonly observed at doses 1.6-6 mg/m^2 I.V. for 30 minutes/week x 4, followed by a two-week rest, resulted in the dose-limiting toxic effects being nausea and vomiting, which were more severe in patients with hepatic metastasis or liver function abnormalities. Other sporadic toxic effects included fever, chills, hypotension, thrombocytosis, and leukocytosis. Hematologic toxicity was insignificant.[40-42]

However, none of the patients who received bruceantin achieved an objective 50 percent tumor regression, but stabilization of disease occurred in some patients at dose levels ≥ 3 mg/m^2. This included patients with colorectal cancer; adenocarinoma of the lung, uterus and cervix; malignant melanoma; and lymphocytic lymphoma. In order for it to be a clinically useful anticancer agent, further research with the aim of potentiating its antitumor activity and decreasing its toxicity is necessary.

3.2 Triptolide derivatives:

The neighboring hydroxyl group may enhance the reactivity of a conjugated ketone toward biological nucleophiles through intramolecular hydrogen bonding, which can activate the unsaturated ketone toward nucleophilic attack by a biological macromolecule.

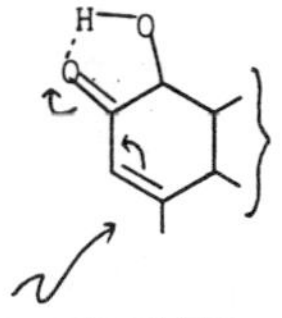

:nucleophile

Fig. 19

Kupchan *et al.*[43] described the inhibition of tumor growth via selective alkylation of the thiol groups of key enzymes involved in growth regulation and the important effect of the hydrogen bond of the alkylation reaction of triptolide derivatives. They are highly active antileukemic principles of the plant *Tripterygium wilfordii* Hook (雷公藤 , *lei-kung t'eng*) of Celastraceae. Triptolide at 0.1 mg/kg showed impressive life-prolonging effects

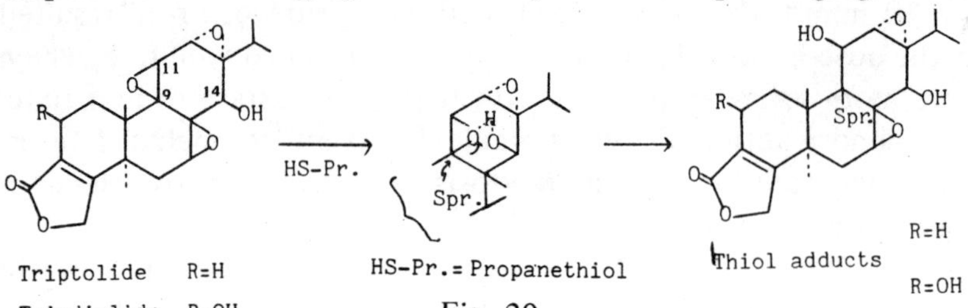

Triptolide R=H
Tripdiolide R=OH

HS-Pr. = Propanethiol

Thiol adducts R=H R=OH

Fig. 20

(T/C > 230) in mice afflicted with L-1210 lymphoid leukemia. Biological and chemical data showed that the $C_{9,11}$-epoxide group was activated by a neighboring C_{14}-β-hydroxy group, making it easily attacked by nucleophiles, such as the –SH group, to form adducts. The thiol adducts (lacking the $C_{9,11}$-epoxide) as well as the minor variants C_{14}-epitriptolide (with an α-OH) and triptonide (lacking the C_{14}-β-OH group) show no antileukemic activity at doses up to 0.4 mg/kg. This indicates the importance of intramolecular interaction for the mode of action of the antileukemic triptolides.

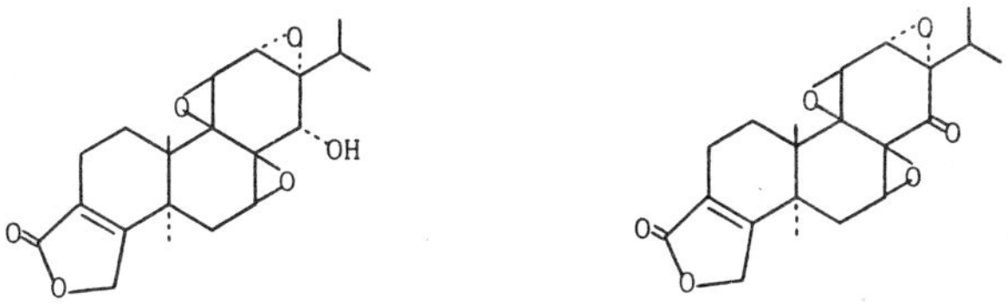

14-Epitriptolide

Triptonide

Fig. 21

3.3 Isodon diterpenoids

Members of the genus *Isodon* (香茶菜屬) of the family Labiatae are perennial herbs growing in mountainous areas. They are widely distributed in southeastern Asia, and have been used as medicinal plants for the treatment of cancer, infections, and other diseases in various countries from ancient times.[44] For example, *I. amethystoides* (香茶菜,王棗子), found in the Yangtze River valley of China, is used in treating lung abscess and myelitis in Chinese medicine.[45] The decocted extract of *I. japonicus* Hara (延命草) or *I. trichocarpus* Kudo has long been used as a local family remedy for gastrointestinal disorders in Japan.[46]

In 1963, Arai *et. al.*[46] reported that the crystalline substances, enmein and enmein-3-acetate obtained from *I. japonicus,* exhibited antitumor activity. A detailed investigation of *Isodon* diterpenoids has been carried out by Fujita *et al.*[46-51] Some more effective antitumor agents, such as oridonin and lasiokaurin have been isolated from *I. japonicus, I. trichocarpus, I. lasiocarpus* (台灣香茶菜) and other *Isodon* species.

Table 14. The Structures of Kaurene Type Diterpenoids from the *Isodon* Genus

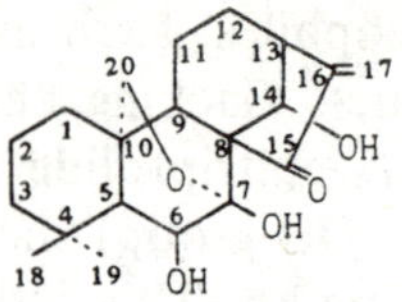

	Compound	Structure	Sources*	References
1.	Oridonin (Rubescensin A)	C_1-OH C_6-OH	1,2,3,4,13	47-51
2.	Ponicidin (Rubescensin B)	C_1-OH $C_{14,20}$-epoxy C_{14}-H	1,4	49
3.	Deoxyoridonin	C_1-OH C_{14}-H	1	47-51
4.	Lasiodonin	C_1-OH C_{11}-OH C_{14}-H	1,2,3	48
5.	Lasiokaurin	C_1-OAc	1,2,3	48
6.	Kamebacetal A	C_1-OH C_{20}-OMe C_6-H	8	52
7.	Kamebacetal B	C_1-OH C_6-H C_{14}-H	8	52
8.	Rubescensin C	C_{11}-OH C_{15}-OH	4	53
9.	Longikaurin A	C_7-H	9,10	54
10.	Longikaurin B	C_7-H C_{19}-CH_2OAc	9,10	54
11.	Trichokaurin	C_1-OH C_{15}-OAc C_{14}-H C_6-OAc	2	50,51

*Sources: 1. *I. japonicus;* 2. *I. trichocarpus;* 3. *I. lasiocarpus;* 4. *I. rubescens;* 5. *I. amethystoides;* 6. *I. japonica* var. *glaucocalyx;* 7. *I. umbrosis;* 8. *I. kameba;* 9. *I. longitubus;* 10. *I. ternifolia;* 11. *I. shikokianus;* 12. *I. obesulus;* 13. *I. macrophyllus;* 14. *Rabdosia shikokiano.*

Table 15. The Structures of Kaurene-type Diterpenoids from the *Isodon* Genus

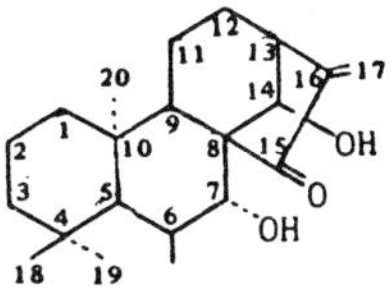

	Compound	Structure	Sources*	Ref.
12.	Umbrosin A	C_2-OH	5,7,8,11	45,55
13.	Umbrosin B	C_2=O	5,7,8,11	55
14.	14-acetylumbrosin B	C_2=O C_{14}-OAc	5,7,8,11	45,55
15.	Isodomedin	C_1-OH C_3-β-OAc	8,11	56
16.	Amethytodin A	C_{11}=O C_{20}-CH_2OH	5	
17.	Wangzaozine A	C_3-OH	5	57
18.	Wangzaozine B (Glaucocalyxin A)	C_3=O	5,6	57
19.	Wangzaozine C (Glaucocalyxin B)	C_3=O C_{14}-OAc	5,6	57
20.	Kamebanin	C_1-OH	8	58
21.	Leukamenin E	C_3-OAc	11,14	59
22.	Shikoccidin	C_9-OH C_3-OAc	11,14	59

*Sources: see Table 14.

Table 16. The Structures of B-seco-kaurene-type Diterpenoids from the *Isodon* genus

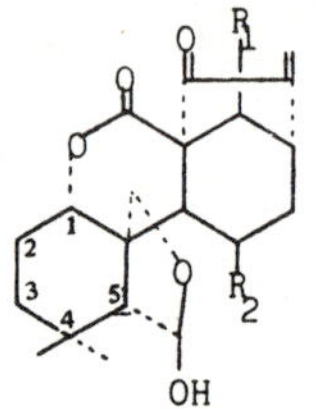

(I)

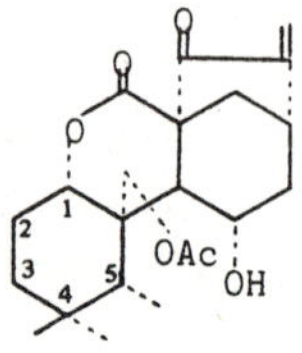

(II)

Compound	Structure	Sources*	References
23. Enmein	(I) C_3-OH R_1=H R_2=H	1,2,3	46
24. Enmein-3-acetate	(I) C_3-OAc R_1=R_2=H	1,2,3	46,60
25. Nodosin	(I) R_1=H R_2=OH	1,2,3	61
26. Isodocarpin	(I) R_1=R_2=H	1,2,3	61
27. Macrophyllin G	(II) C_5-CH_2OH	13	
28. Isodonoic acid	(II) C_5-COOH	10	54
29. Isodonal	(II) C_5-CHO	10,13	54,62

*Sources: see Table 14

Subsequently, more compounds of this class have been reported as shown in Tables 14, 15, and 16.

In China, researchers isolated oridonin and ponicidin from *I. rubescens* (冬淩草) and used them for the treatment of esophageal and cardial carcinoma in clinical trials.[63-65] In addition, some other *Isodon* diterpenoids also exhibited antitumor activity *in vitro* and/or *in vivo* in varying degrees. Therefore, considerable attention has been given to *Isodon* plants.

Based on the carbon skeleton and functionalities, the diterpenoids from plants of the *Isodon* genus can be classified into kaurenes and B-seco-kaurenes. In view of the facts that tricho-

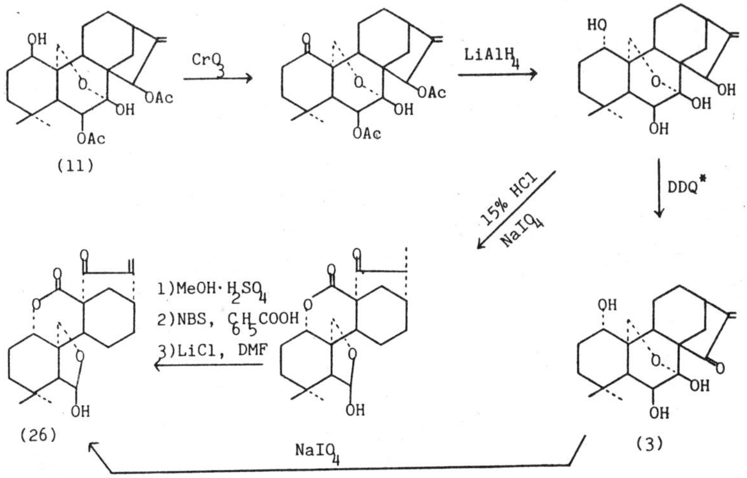

(11) $\xrightarrow{CrO_3}$ $\xrightarrow{LiAlH_4}$ $\xrightarrow{DDQ^*}$ (3)

$\xrightarrow{15\%\ HCl,\ NaIO_4}$ $\xrightarrow{1)\ MeOH\cdot H_2SO_4;\ 2)\ NBS,\ C_6H_5COOH;\ 3)\ LiCl,\ DMF}$ (26)

(3) $\xrightarrow{NaIO_4}$ (26)

*DDQ: 2,3-dichloro-5,6-dicyano-1,4-benzoquinone

Fig. 22

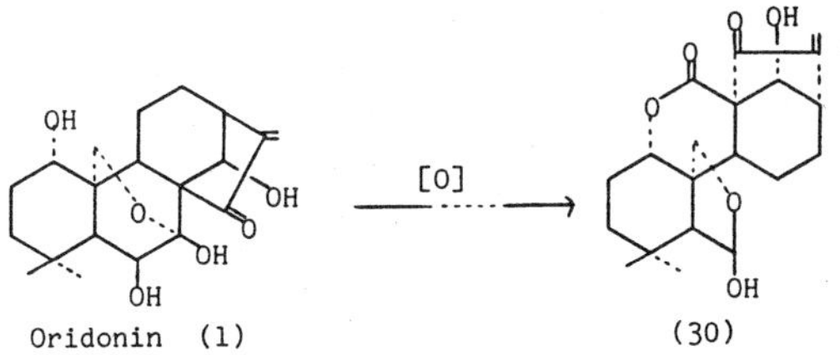

Oridonin (1) $\xrightarrow{[O]}$ (30)

Fig. 23

kaurin and oridonin, kaurenoids isolated from *I. trichocarpus*, have been chemically converted into their corresponding B-seco-kaurene derivatives,[66] and that ent-kaur-16-ene and ent-kaur-16-en-15-one were shown to be precursors of enmein and oridonin by feeding 7-ent-kaur-16-ene-17-C^{14} derivatives to growing *I. japonicus* plants,[67] it is thought that the B-seco-kaurene type diterpenoid is biogenetically derived from (–)- kaurene by oxidative cleavage of its B-ring, followed by recyclization.

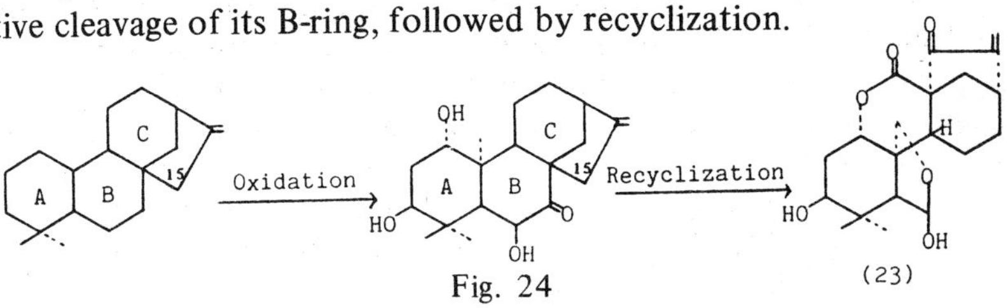

$\xrightarrow{Oxidation}$ $\xrightarrow{Recyclization}$ (23)

Fig. 24

Functionalization of the C-15 position proceeds though direct oxidation.

Most of these compounds from the *Isodon* genus contain α-methylene-cyclo-pentanone, a highly electrophilic conjugated system. This portion of the molecule is thought to play an important role in interaction with biological nucleophiles and in the mechanism of their antitumor activity. In the Michael-type additions of model biological nucleophiles to α-methylenecyclopentanone system of *Isodon* diterpenoids, oridonin easily reacted with thiols and L-cysteine to yield thiol adduct 32 under mild conditions.[50]

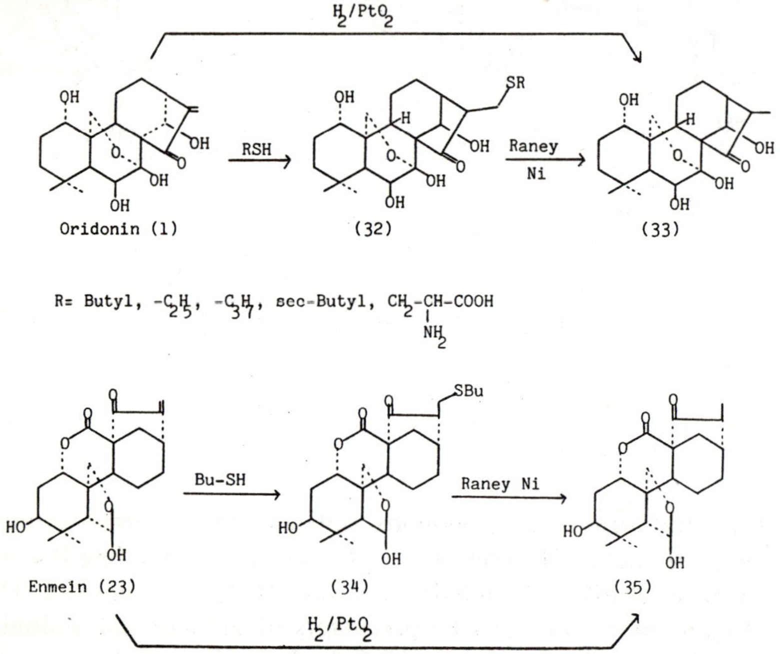

H_2/PtO_2

RSH → Raney Ni →

Oridonin (1) (32) (33)

R= Butyl, $-C_2H_5$, $-C_3H_7$, sec-Butyl, CH_2-CH(NH_2)-COOH

Bu-SH → Raney Ni →

Enmein (23) (34) (35)

H_2/PtO_2

Fig. 25

Enmein also easily yielded adduct 34 by reaction with butane thiol, although its reactivity is lower than that of oridonin.

The presence of a hydrogen bond between the carbonyl group at the C-15 position and the hydroxy group at the C-6 position in the oridonin molecule has been confirmed by its IR, UV, and NMR spectra[47] (see Table 16). Therefore, the C-17 atom is polarized, giving a positive center and thus increasing its reactivity with the nucleophile.

Table 17. The C-17 Proton Chemical Shifts of Oridonin, Enmein, and Its Derivatives in Their NMR Spectra

Compound	Chemical shifts of methylene protons of C-17 (δ PPm)	
Oridonin (1)	5.53	6.31
Rubescensin C (8)	5.16	5.21
Enmein (23)	5.43	5.98
Enmein-3-acetate (24)	5.33	5.99
Compound (30)	5.40	6.12

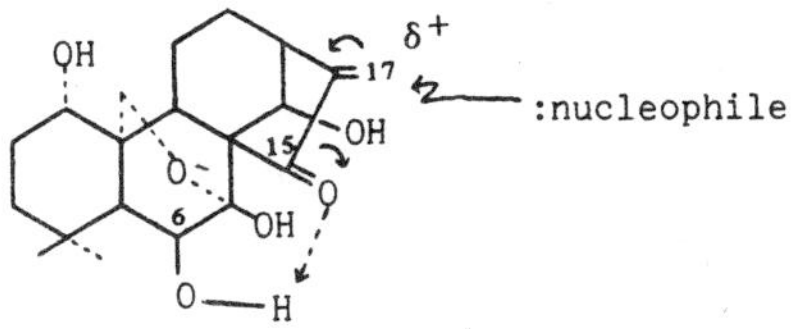

Fig. 26

Since the antitumor activities of many tumor inhibitors having hydroxyl groups are often enhanced by acylation of the hydroxyl groups, Nagao *et al.*[68,69] studied the selective acylation of hydroxyl groups in the oridonin molecule.

The oxygen atom of the C-6-OH has the strongest nucleophilicity because of the hydrogen bonding with C-15 carbonyl group, using $(RCO)_2O$ as the acylating reagent in the pyridine resulted only in C-14-esters.[36-43] In an $(RCO)_2O$-catalytic $BF_3 \cdot EtO_2$ reagent system, however, acid anhydride may be activated by BF_3 to an active species, which more easily acylates the hydroxyl group at C-6 position.

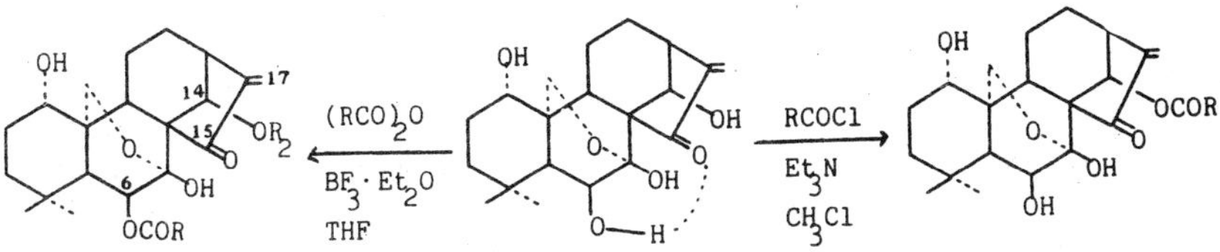

Fig. 27

As the carbon atom at the C-17 position is expected to be polarized by hydrogen bonding between C-6-OH and C-15 = O, and to increase the reactivity with the nucleophilic agents, it is not surprising that C-6-O-acyl derivatives (44-46) of oridonin have no antitumor activity, but the activity of C-14-O-acyl derivatives increased with the increased acyl carbon chain length (Table 18), indicating that the ester side chain in oridonin C-14-O-acyl derivatives (36-43) may play a carrier role in the processes related to cell penetration.

Table 18. Antitumor Activity of Oridonin and Its C-6-acyl (36-43) and C-14-acyl (44-46) Derivatives Against Ehrlich Ascites Carcinoma in Mice

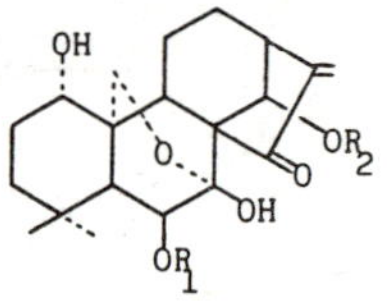

OH
OR_2
O
O
OH
OR_1

Compound	Structure	T/C %	(mg/kg)
Oridonin	R_1=R_2=H	125.5	(5.0)
		142.6	(10.0)
36	R_1=H R_2=COPh	124.0	(5.0)
		158.2	(10.0)
37	R_1=H R_2=COCH=CHPh	127.0	(5.0)
		103	(10.0)
38	R_1=H R_2=COC_3H_7	117	(10.0)
39	R_1=H R_2=COC_5H_{11}	132	(5.0)
		123	(10.0)
40	R_1=H R_2=COC_9H_{19}	136.9	(5.0)
		135	(10.0)
41	R_1=H R_2=$COC_{11}H_{23}$	142.6	(5.0)
		141.8	(10.0)
42	R_1=H R_2=$COC_{13}H_{27}$	156.7	(5.0)
		161.0	(10.0)
43	R_1=H R_2=$COC_{15}H_{31}$	176.6	(5.0)
		190.0	(10.0)
44	R_1=Ac R_2=H	102.3	(5.0)
		113	(10.0)
45	R_1=R_2=Ac	106.9	(5.0)
		109	(10.0)
46	R_1=$COC_{11}H_{23}$ R_2=H	69	(5.0)
		101	(10.0)

Antitumor action:

Arai *et al.*[46] reported that enmein and its diacetate possessed antitumor activity, while dihydroenmein remained inactive. The exocyclic methylene group attached to five-membered cyclic ketone in enmein proves essential to this biological activity.

Fujita *et al.*[50,51] investigated in detail the antitumor activity of oridonin, lasiokaurin, enmein, and related compounds against Ehrlich ascites carcinoma by injecting 5 to 40 mg/kg of these compounds every 24 hours after the tumor was inoculated in mice for seven days, followed by observation for 33 days. The results are summarized in Table 19.

Table 19. Antitumor Activity of *Isodon* Diterpenoids and Related Compounds Against Ehrlich Ascites Carcinoma in Mice

Compound	Dose (mg/kg)	ILS*%
Oridonin	10	115
Lasiokaurin	10	117
Trichokurin	10	17
Enmein	10	39
	25	66
	40	86
Compound (33)	10	9
Compound (30)	10	4
Deoxyoridonin	10	24
	20	61
Compound (32)	10	7

*ILS: Increase of lifespan.

Oridonin and lasiokaurin showed significant activity, while enmein, enmein-3-acetate, and compound 30 derived from oridonin showed activity at a higher dose than that of oridonin. Both the $\Delta^{16,17}$ saturated derivatives (compounds 33, 35) and n-butane thiol adducts (compounds 32, 34) did not show any activity. Trichokaurin, lacking a carbonyl group at the C-15 position, showed no antitumor activity. These facts suggest that the α-methylene cyclopentanone function is the important active center for the activity of these compounds. The activities of C-14 deoxyoridonin, as well as enmein, enmein-3-acetate, and compound 30, are 1/4 or less of that of oridonin, reflecting that some hydroxyl groups present at a position suitable for contact with and binding with an enzyme containing a specific nucleophile are also necessary for the activity. A hydrogen bonding between the C-6-OH group and the carbonyl group at the C-15 position is especially important for enhancing the electrophilicity of the carbon atom at the C-17 position. The mode of action of oridonin has been suggested by Fujita *et al.* as follows:[50,51]

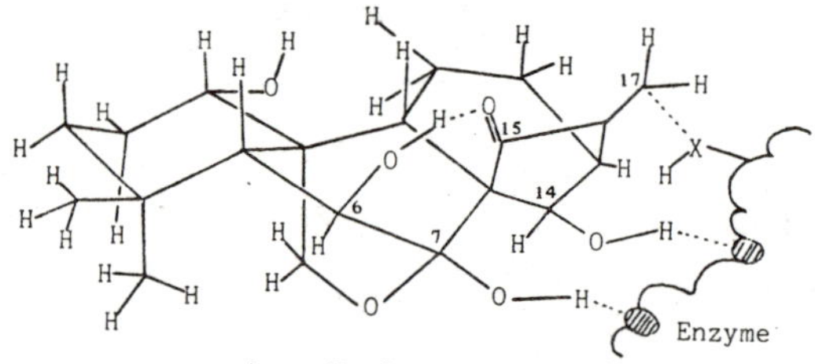

where X= S or NH

Fig. 28

Recently, Nagao *et al.*[70] further reported on the tumor-inhibitory test of *Isodon* diterpenoids against P-388 lymphocytic leukemia in mice (see Table 20). The results showed that *Isodon* diterpenoids possess considerable activity against P-388 lymphocytic leukemia, as in the case of activity against Ehrlich ascites carcinoma. In the P-388 system oridonin and enmein showed similar activities, but the hydrogen bonding in oridonin seems not to enhance the antitumor activity in the P-388 system.

Shikoccin, possessing an unique 8,9-seco-kaurene skeleton, was isolated from *Rabdosia shikokiano*. It also showed significant activity against P-388 lymphocytic leukemia.[59,70]

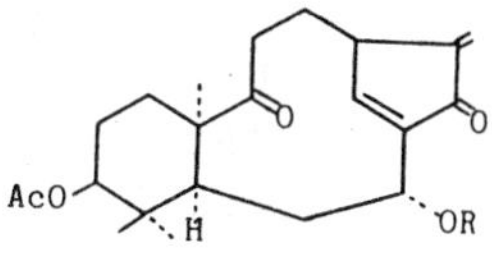

AcO H OR

Shikoccin R=H

Methylshikoccin R=Me

Fig. 29

In addition, wangzaozine B, isolated from *I. japonica* var. *glaucocalyx* (藍萼香茶菜) and *I. amthystoides* (王棗子), has been reported to be effective against sarcoma-180 and Ehrlich ascites carcinoma.

Table 20. Antitumor Activity of *Isodon* Diterpenoids Against P-388 Lymphocytic Leukemia

Compound	Dose (mg/kg)	Optimum T/C*%
Oridonin	12.0	127
	18.0	131
Enmein	12.5	125
	25.0	137
Enmein-3-acetate	10.0	124
Nodosin	5.0	120
	40.0	124
Shikoccin	15.0	123
	50.0	124

*T/C = mean survival days (treated)/mean survival days (control).

Macrophyllin G, a new diterpenoid derived from *I. macrophyllus* (大葉香茶菜), also very significantly increased lifespan in animal tumor experiments.[5]

Recently, Fujita *et al.*[72] isolated longikaurin A and B from *I. longitubus* (長管香茶菜). The former exhibited *in vitro* inhibitory action against breast cancer FM3/4 in mice.

Another new diterpenoid, shikodonin, having an unique spiro-seco-kaurene structure was isolated from the dry leaves of *I. shikokianus* along with oridonin and shikokianin. Shikodonin possessed significant *in vitro* cytotoxicity (KB) and *in vivo* anti-tumor activity against Ehrlich ascites carcinoma in mice. It also exhibited insect growth inhibitory activity, specifically against *Lepidoptera* larvae.[73]

Wedeloside and its L-rhamnopyranosyl glycoside isolated from *Wedelia asperrima* Benth. (Compositae) are the very rare examples of an amino sugar occurring in plants. Preliminary experiments with rats suggests that wedeloside has an inhibiting effect on tumors produced by aflatoxin B.[74]

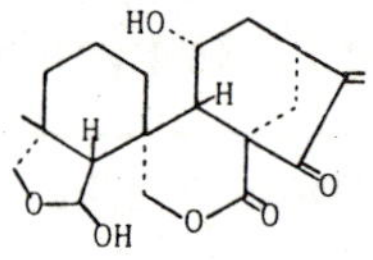

Shikodonin

Table 21. Cytotoxicity of *Isodon* Diterpenoids *in vitro* Against KB Cells

Compound	ID_{50} (μg/ml)
Oridonin	2.8
Isodomedin	4.0
Shikodonin	4.2
Shikokianin	10.0

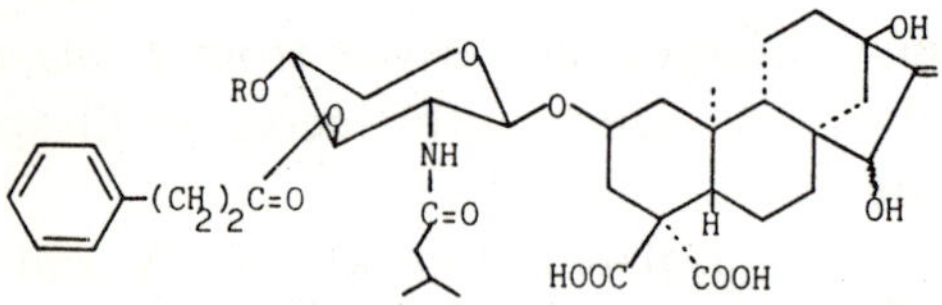

Wedeloside
R=H
Wedeloside glycoside
R = L-rhamnopyranosyl

Fig. 30

Antibacterial activity

Early reports on the antibacterial activity of *Isodon* diterpenoids by Arai *et al.* and Kubo *et al.*[75] indicated that oridonin exhibited a moderate inhibitory activity against nineteen kinds of bacteria, specifically gram-positive bacteria. Lasiodonin, deoxyoridonin, enmein, and enmein-3-acetate also showed activity against gram-positive bacteria, while $\Delta^{16,17}$ saturated derivatives, thiol adducts, and trichokaurin lacking the C-15 carbonyl group did not have any activity. On the other hand, the antibacterial activity of oridonin, lasiodonin, and deoxyoridonin was higher than that of enmein and enmein-3-acetate. These findings also indicated that the active center was the α-methylene-cyclopentanone function. A hydrogen bonding between the C-6-hydroxy group and the C-15-carbonyl group played an important role in increased activity.

On the mechanism of action of *Isodon* diterpenoids, it has been shown that some inhibited oxidative phosphorylation and significantly depressed the rate of respiration in mitochondria.[76] (See Table 22).

Table 22. Effect of Isodon Diterpenoids on the Energy-linked Functions of Mitochondria from Termite Queen Ovaries

Compound	Concentration (μm)	Respiratory Control Ratio	Phosphorylation Rate
Oridonin	100	3.63	156
Isodonal	100	2.66	122
Enmein	100	3.41	181
Nodosin	250	2.30	170
Control	–	4.43	256

The inhibition of these biochemical parameters may result from their reaction with the essential -SH group of the enzymes involved in these processes.

3.4 Daphnane diterpene ester

Compounds belonging to the daphnane diterpene esters, such as gnidilatidin isolated from *Daphne genkwa* (芫花 , *yan-hua*) and *D. odorata* (瑞香, *sue-shiang*) of the Thymelaeaceae (瑞香科), have previously been shown to have antileukemic activity as opposed to tigliane diterpene esters, for example, phorbol esters, found in the genus *Croton* (Euphorbiaceae), which are known to be tumor-promoting agents. Some plants of the *Daphne* or *Gnidia* genus of the same family have historically been used in herbal medicine to treat human cancer and warts. Some antileukemic *Daphne* esters, such as gnidimacrin and its C-20 palmitate, have been isolated from *Gnidia* plants of the family. Some investigators suggest that the C-20 and C-12 ester groups are necessary for antileukemic activity, and that these groups enable the agent to pass through the cellular membranes, thus facilitating its antineoplastic effect.[77]

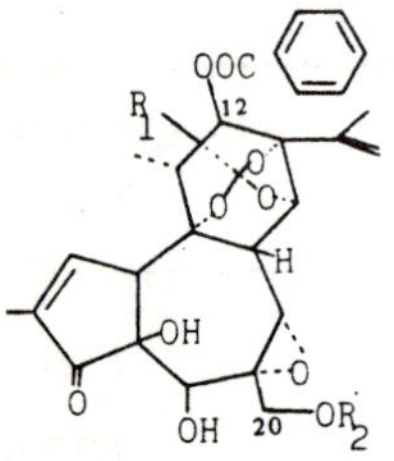

Gnidilatidin R_1=CH=CH-CH=CH-$(CH_2)_3CH_3$
R_2=H

Gnidilatidin-20-palmitate R_1=CH=CH-CH=CH-$(CH_2)_4CH_3$
R_2=$COC_{15}H_{31}$

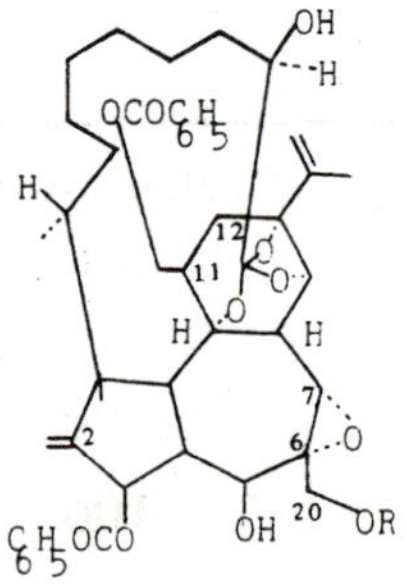

Gnidimacrin R=H

Gnidimacrin-20-palmitate R=$COC_{15}H_{31}$

Fig. 31

Daphnane diterpenoids are highly oxygenated diterpenoids and contain an α, β-unsaturated cyclopentenone. Gnidimacrin and its 20-palmitate ester contain a novel macrocyclic ring with a terminus at the ortho ester carbon. The significance of these structural features as well as the C-6, C-7 epoxide has not yet been established.[78]

Table 23. Activity of Daphnane Diterpenoids Against P-388 Lymphocytic Leukemia in Mice

Compound	T/C (in P-388) %
Gnidilatidin	140 at 0.5 mg/kg
Gnidilatidin-20-palmitate	170 at 0.5 mg/kg
Gnidimacrin	180 at 12-16 μg/kg
Gnidimacrin-20-palmitate	190 at 30-50 μg/kg

4. Triterpenes

4.1 Cardenolides

The milkweeds of the genus *Asclepias* (Asclepiadaceae) are well known for their folkloric uses in the treatment of many cancerous states. Some years ago, calotropin was isolated and identified as the major cytotoxic principle of *Asclepias curassavica* (馬利筋 , *ma-li-gen*).

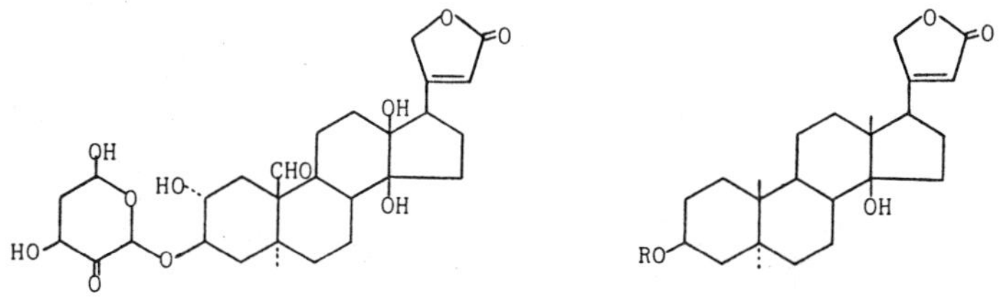

Calotropin

Uzarigenin R=H

Desglucouzarin R=β-D-glucopyranosyl

Fig. 32

Recently, Koike *et al.*[79] examined extracts of the California plant *A. albicans* S. Wats. A 50% aqueous ethanol extract of *A. albicans* showed consistent activity on the carcinoma of the nasopharynx (KB) test system in cell cultures. The cytotoxic activity of extracts of *A. albicans* was traced to uzarigenin and its glucoside, which are well-established constituents of several *Asclepias* species, such as *A. curassavica, A. glaucophylla,* and *A. lilacina.*

The previously known cytotoxic cardenolides, strophanthidin and its glucoside, having an $ED_{50} < 0.25$ μg/ml in cell cultures against carcinoma of the nasopharynx, were isolated from *Adonis amurensis* (Ranunculaceae) (福壽草 , *xu-sou cao*).[80]

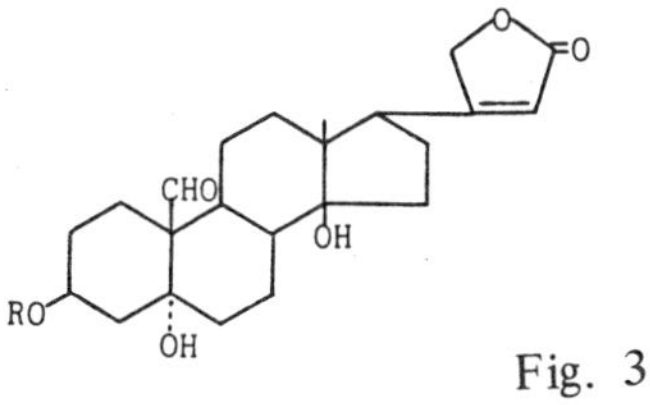

Strophanthidin R=H

Strophanthidin glucoside R=Glu.

Fig. 33

These cytotoxic and antitumor cardenolides have a steroid ring structure as well as a five-membered α, β-unsaturated lactone function.

4.2 Cucurbitacins

Cucurbitacins are triterpenoids possessing cytotoxic and/or antitumor activity. They are widely present in several medicinal plants of Cucurbitaceae, Cruciferae, Scrophulariaceae, and Begoniaceae. These compounds exhibit exceptionally high cytotoxicity in tissue culture tests on KB and HeLa cells.[81-84]

The common characteristics of these compounds are an α-hydroxy ketone in ring A and carbonyl at C-11 and C-22, the latter being conjugated to a $\Delta^{23,24}$ double bond. Some members also contain a $\Delta^{5,6}$ or $\Delta^{6,7}$ double bond in their structure.

The cytotoxic and antitumor activity *in vivo* depends on the existence of a double bond in the side chain of these compounds. Saturation of the conjugated $\Delta^{23,24}$ double bond in cucurbitacins is accompanied by a profound lessening in cytotoxicity of the resultant dihydrocucurbitacin. As shown below, reaction of the side-chain conjugated ketone with biological macromolecules may play an important role in the mechanism by which cucurbitacins exert their cytotoxic effect. The acetylation of the C-16-OH group of cucurbitacin B produced fabacein with marked diminution of cytotoxity, suggesting the hydrogen-bonding interaction between the C-16-OH group and that the C-22 ketone could activate the α, β-unsaturated ketone system toward nucleophilic attack by a biological macromolecule.[81]

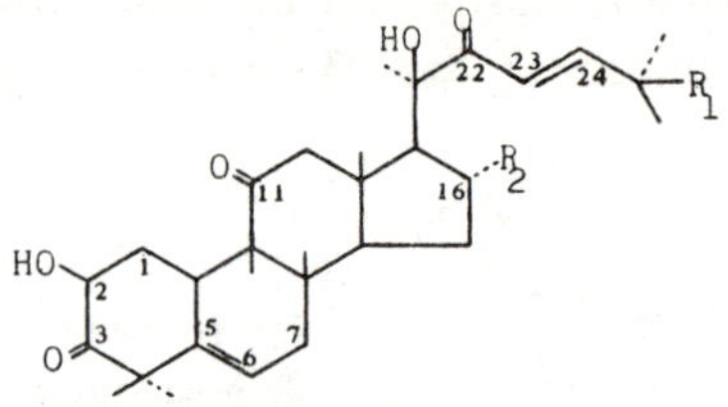

Fig. 34

	R_1	R_2	Others
Cucurbitacin B	OAc	OH	
Fabacein	OAc	OAc	
Cucurbitacin D	OH	OH	
Cucurbitacin E	OH	OH	$\Delta^{1,2}$
Cucurbitacin L	OAc	OH	$\Delta^{1,2}$ $C_{23\text{-}24}$ hydrogenation

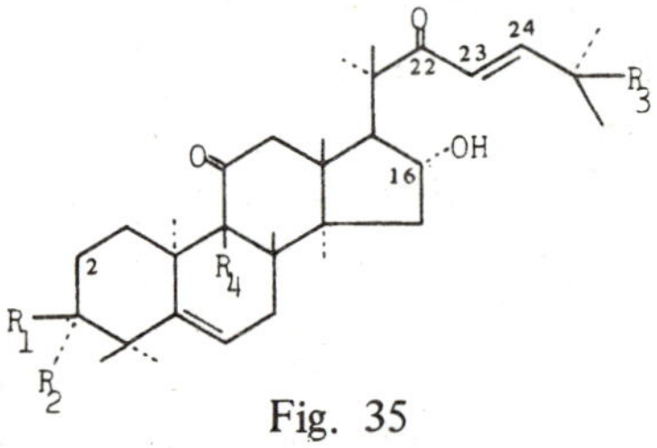

Fig. 35

	R_1	R_2	R_3	R_4	Others
Cucurbitacin C	OH	H	OAc	CH_2OH	
Isocucurbitacin D	H	OH	OH	CH_3	C = O

Table 24. Cytotoxicity and Antitumor Activity of Cucurbitacins

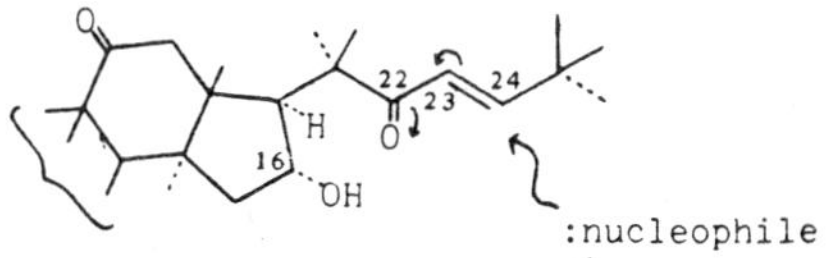

Fig. 36

Compounds	ED_{50} μg/ml KB	HeLa Cell	Other
Cucurbitacin B	2.5×10^{-6}	0.005	
Cucurbitacin C	0.001		
Cucurbitacin D	0.005-0.01	0.01-0.05	S-180
Cucurbitacin E	0.01	0.01-0.05	S-180, Lewis lung carcinoma
Cucurbitacin L	0.01-0.1	0.1-0.5	
Isocucurbitacin D	0.024	0.01-0.05	WM-256
Dihydrocucurbitacin B	0.0017		
Fabacein	1.0		

Although cucurbitacins possess a very high order of cytotoxicity, the low antitumor activity *in vivo* and the low margins between effective and toxic doses render the materials unpromising as therapeutic agents. However, they might be interesting subjects for the preparation of semisynthetic derivatives with improved pharmacological properties.

5. Quinones

The benzoquinol jacaranone isolated from *Jacaranda caucana* Pittier (Bignoniaceae)[85-87] and the related ethyl ester isolated from another plant, *Senecio fendeleri* Gray[88-89] (Compositae) possess relatively high biological activity (Ps T/C = 165 at 2 mg/kg), which led to the synthesis of naphthoquinols.

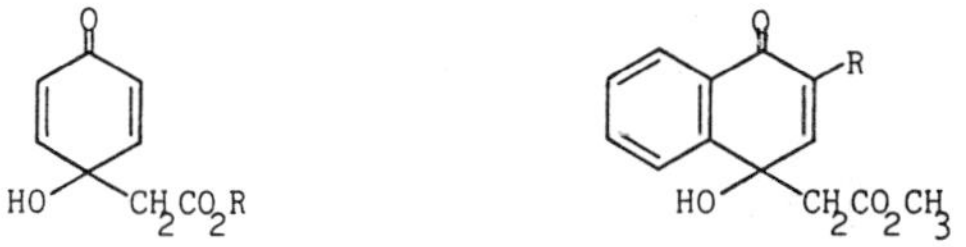

Jacaranone $R = CH_3$ $R = H, OCH_3, CH_3$

Fig. 37

All of these naphthoquinols were screened for cytotoxicity in the KB *in vitro* test system, but none of the compounds was as active ($ED_{50} > 4$ µg/ml) as jacaranone and its ethyl ester homologs. Possibly the requirements for activity in this γ-hydroxy-α, β-unsaturated enone system involve the lack of substitution at either α, β double bond, the most reactive system possible for conjugate addition.[90]

However, the furonaphthoquinones isolated from *Tabebuia cassinoides* (Bignoniaceae), showed slight but reproducible activity in the P-388 *in vivo* bioassay (T/C = 127 and 125 at 200 mg/kg in two separate tests).[91]

KB ED_{50} = 1.0 µg/ml ED_{50} = 2.0 µg/ml

Fig. 38

Both compounds show significant activity in the KB cell culture (ED_{50} = 1.0 and 2.0 μg/ml, respectively). The statement has been made that in the quinone series, activity against KB cells at levels less than 1 μg/ml appears to correlate with activity in the L-1210 lymphoid leukemia system *in vivo.*[92]

On the other hand, the occurrence of naphthoquinones in various members of the genus *Tabebuia* is well known, and lapachol is one of the major constituents of several *Tabebuia* species, *Stereospermum suareolens* (羽葉楸), *Tecoma* (Bignoniaceae), *Avicennia officinalis* (Verbenaceae) (海欖雌) and *Bassia latifolia* (Chenopodiaceae). Lapachol exhibited significant inhibitory activity against WM-256, Ehrlich ascites carcinoma, and lymphoma MS. In the tumor-inhibitory tests against WM-256, 99% inhibition was reached[93] so that NCI[92] began clinical trials even though the ED_{50} value of this compound in KB cell culture was 4.4 μg/ml.

The biosynthesis of furonaphthoquinone may occur via cyclization of lapachol.[91]

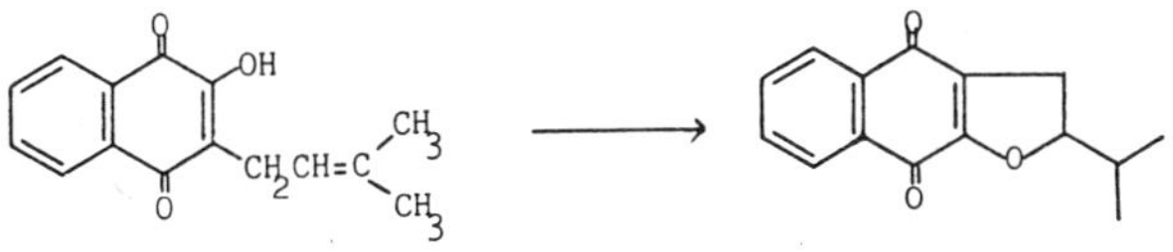

Lapachol

(KB ED_{50} = 4.4 μg/ml)

Fig. 39

Other naphthoquinones, shikonin and its derivatives contained in the root of *Lithospermum officinalis* var. *erythrorhizon* Max. and *Macrogtomia enchroma* (紫草) (Boraginaceae) also showed high antitumor activity against the ascites cells of S-180, and WM-256. Shikonin completely inhibited S-180 carcinoma growth at a dose of 5-15 mg/kg/day, but was inactive against L-1210. However, the structural similarity of shikonin to daunomycin and adriamycin suggests that it may be possible to prepare more active compounds by further functionalization.[94,95]

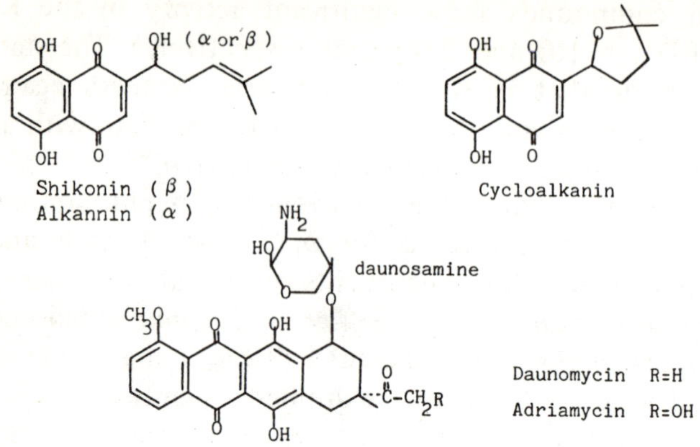
OH (α or β)
Shikonin (β)
Alkannin (α)
Cycloalkanin
daunosamine
Daunomycin R=H
Adriamycin R=OH

Fig. 40

Taxodone and taxodione isolated from *Taxodium distichum* (落羽杉) demonstrated significant inhibitory activity against WM-256 in rats at 40 and 25 mg/kg dose levels.[96,97]

Taxodione Taxodone

Fig. 41

Under very mild conditions, addition of ammonia to taxodione readily gives a purple-colored crystalline product; the reaction can be visualized as having proceeded via the Michael addition. Similarly, the Michael addition on C-7 position with biological nucleophiles may be the mechanism of their activity.[13,96]

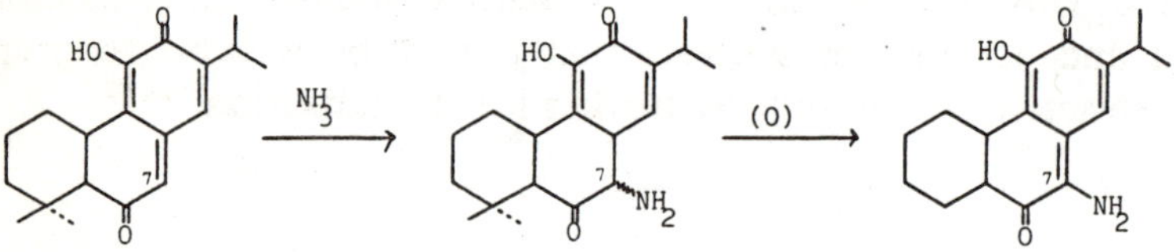
NH3
(O)

Fig. 42

Barbatusin, isolated from *Coleus barbutus* (Labiatae), possessed significant inhibitory activity against Lewis lung carcinoma and lymphocytic leukemia P-388 in mice at dose levels of 200 and 400 mg/kg.[98]

Barbatusin

Fig. 43

In addition, przewaquinone A and B contained in *Salvia przewalskii* var. *mandarinorum* (紫丹參),[99] irisquinone isolated from *Iris pallasii* var. *chinensis* (馬藺子), and juglone isolated from *Juglans nigra* (黑胡桃) (Juglandaceae) all possess considerable antitumor activity.

Przewaquinone A

Przewaquinone B

Irisquinone

Juglone

Fig. 44

Schwenk[100] tested a number of natural and synthetic substances with quinone, methylenequinone, and iminoquinone structures on the cheekpouch tumor of the golden hamster. A

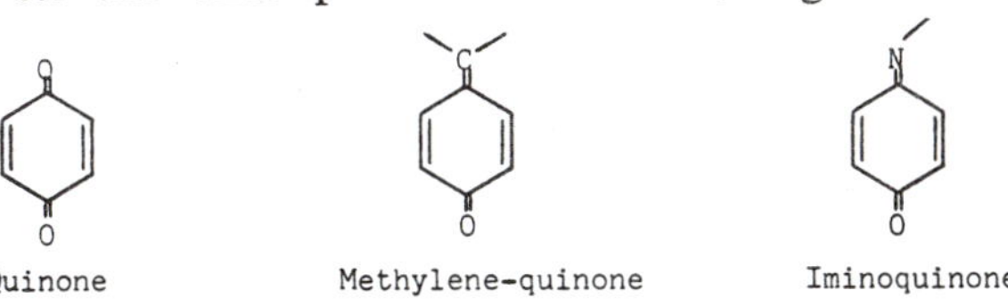

Fig. 45

possible connection between the tumor growth and the hydrogen peroxide formation was suggested: The anthraquinones are catalytically reduced by hydrogen to anthrahydroquinones, which in the presence of traces of water with molecular oxygen from air revert to the starting anthraquinone, and give nearly pure hydrogen peroxide which interferes with the growth of tumor cells by inhibiting their glycolysis.

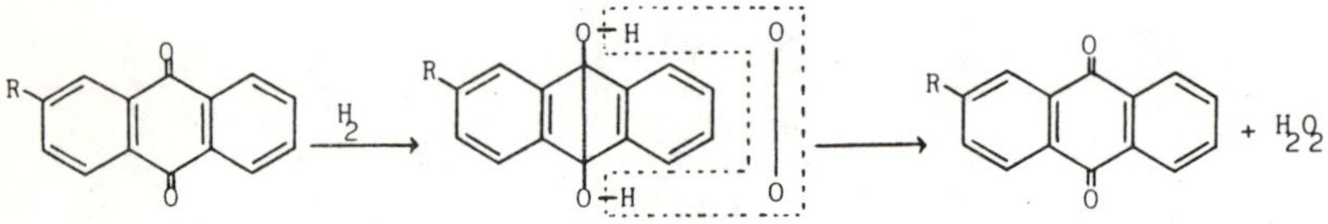

Fig. 46

The methanolic extract of the rhizome and root of *Morinda parvifolia* Bart (*bai-yan-teng* 百眼藤) (Rubiaceae) showed significant inhibitory activity *in vivo* against P-388 growth in mice (T/C = 152%) at 50 mg/kg/day, I.P. Bioassay directed toward isolation of the antileukemic principle recently led to the characterization of morindaparin A, a new cytotoxic and antileukemic anthraquinone, with an ED_{50} = 1.85 μg/ml against the *in vitro* growth of P-388 lymphocytic leukemia in tissue culture.[101]

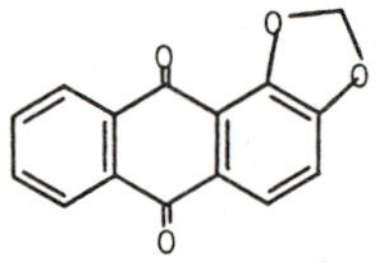

Morindaparin A

Fig. 47

Since alizarin (I) gave a significant antileukemic activity with a T/C = 134% at 10 mg/kg, its esters such as the acetates (VI, VII) the cinnamates (VIII, IX), and the senecioates (X, XI) were prepared by general methods for possible enhancement of the *in vivo* antileukemic activity. However, these esters lack *in vivo* antileukemic activity, probably due to supraoptimum lipophilicity and/or insufficient water solubility.

Table 25. Antitumor Activity of Alizarin and Its Derivatives Against P-388 Lymphocytic Leukemia

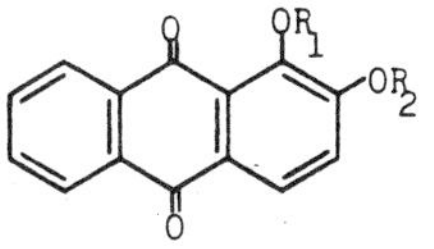

No.	Structure	T/C % (dose)
I.	$R_1 = R_2 = H$	134 (10 mg/kg)
II.	$R_1 = Me \quad R_2 = H$	136 (10 mg/kg)
III.	$R_1 = H \quad R_2 = Me$	126 (10.0)
IV.	$R_1 R_2 = -CH_2CH_2-$	130 (10.0)
V.	$R_1 R_2 = -CH_2-$	129 (10.0)
VI.	$R_1 = H \quad R_2 = COMe$	
VII.	$R_1 = R_2 = COMe$	
VIII.	$R_1 = H \quad R_2 = CO\text{-}CH{=}CH\text{-}C_6H_5$ 	
IX.	$R_1 = R_2 = -CO\text{-}CH{=}CH\text{-}C_6H_5$	
X.	$R_1 = H \quad R_2 = -COCH = C(Me)_2$	
XI.	$R_1 = R_2 = -COCH = C(Me)_2$	

6. Podophyllotoxins

Podophyllotoxin and its derivatives, present in some plants of the genus *Podophyllum* (Berberidaceae) and the Burseraceae, are known to possess antitumor activity. They produce metaphase arrest and have a mode of action similar to the other spindle poisons, such as colchicine and the vinca alkaloids.

The inhibitory activity of these compounds on microtubule assembly is sensitive to the configuration and size of substituents at position 4 in ring C. But as an antitumor agent, podophyllotoxin itself is too toxic to be useful in man,[102] although it and β-peltatin have the greatest activity in several transplantable rodent tumors.

Podophyllotoxins possess a unique absolute configuration as (1R, 2R, 3R, 4R) with a highly strained, transfused γ-lactone system. This is closely associated with their antimitotic and antitumor activity. By base catalysis podophyllotoxin can be smoothly converted to the more stable cis-fused form, picropodophyllotoxin, which shows little or no cytotoxic activity like its open lactone derivatives.

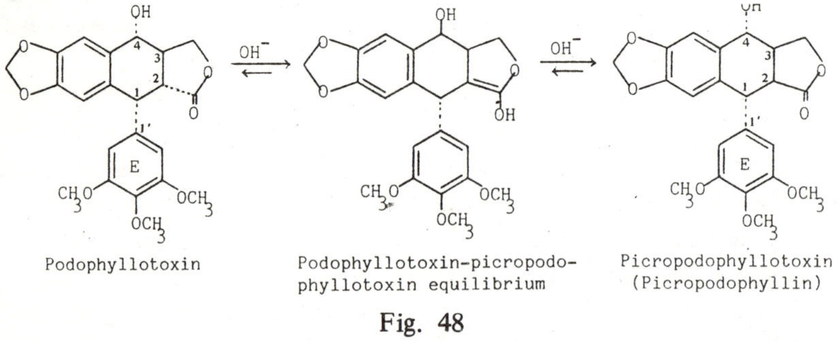

Podophyllotoxin

Podophyllotoxin-picropodophyllotoxin equilibrium

Picropodophyllotoxin (Picropodophyllin)

Fig. 48

Table 26. Structures of Podophyllotoxins and Their Inhibitory Activity on Microtubule Assembly

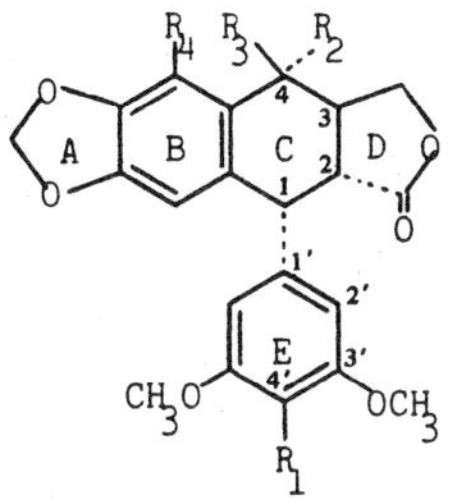

Compound	Structure R_1	R_2	R_3	R_4	ID_{50} (μM)
Podophyllotoxin	OCH_3	OH	H	H	0.6
Epipodophyllotoxin	OCH_3	H	OH	H	5.0
Desoxypodophyllotoxin	OCH_3	H	H	H	0.5
β-Peltatin	OCH_3	H	H	OH	0.7
4'-Demethylpodo-phyllotoxin	OH	OH	H	OH	0.5
4'-Demethylepipodo-phyllotoxin	OH	H	OH	H	2.0
4'-Demethyldeoxypodo-phyllotoxin	OH	H	H	H	0.2
VM-26	OH	H	Thenylidene glucoside	H	–
VP-16	OH	H	Ethylene glucoside	H	–

In podophyllotoxin, the ring E cannot rotate entirely freely because of steric crowding, and it flips down into a quasi-axial position, which may be the active conformation for binding with tubulin. Whereas in picropodophyllotoxin this group can rotate freely about the C-1'-C-1 bond, the active conformation being present in only a small percentage.

This conversion is thought to occur under physiological conditions and constitutes a detoxification of podophyllotoxin.

The C_4-isomers, epipodophyllotoxins, are less active than podophyllotoxins, indicating that there is geometric constraint on the C-4 position at the receptor site, which may have unfavorable interaction between tubulin and the hydroxy group of epipodophyllotoxin.

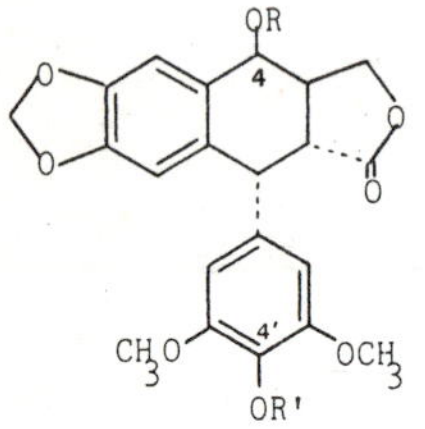

Epipodophyllotoxin R=H R′=CH_3
4′-Demethylepipodophyllotoxin R=R′=H
Epipodophyllotoxin β-D-glucopyranoside
R=β-D-glucopyranoside R′=CH_3
4′-Demethylepipodophyllotoxin β-D-glucopyranoside
R=β-D-glucopyranoside R′=H

Fig. 49

The glucosides of podophyllotoxin, β-peltatin and 4'-demethylpodophyllotoxin were found to be 10^2 -10^4 times less active than their corresponding aglycones in inhibiting the growth of cell cultures and experimentally induced tumors in mice by stopping cell division in early metaphase. Against Ehrlich murine ascites tumors they were five to ten times less active and had less noxious side effects. This information suggests that hydrophilicity and bulk of the glucopyranoside group decrease tubulin binding considerably.

When the glucose residue was partially substituted by condensation with various aldehydes, some compounds were found to have considerable antitumor activity *in vitro*, comparable to that of podophyllotoxin, and remarkably low toxic side effects. They are not only well absorbed by the intestinal tract as podophyllotoxin glucoside, but have an increased lifetime in the body.

Conversion of the C-4' methoxyl group of podophyllotoxin to a hydroxyl group results in only slight decrease in activity. Aldehyde condensation products of 4'-demethylpodophyllotoxin β-D-glucopyranoside were also found to have a pronounced increase in antimitotic effects in experimental animals when administered in well-tolerated doses, and only a few toxic side effects were noticed. The cyclic acetals of epipodophyllotoxin β-D-glucopyranoside revealed no dramatic increase in biological activity. However, some cyclic acetals and ketals of 4'-demethylepipodophyllotoxin β-D-glucopyranoside not only exhibited high activity *in vitro*, but also gave a significant survival time increase in L-1210 lymphoid leukemia test. VM-26 and VP-16 are the best in this series, and quickly entered clinical trials.[102-107]

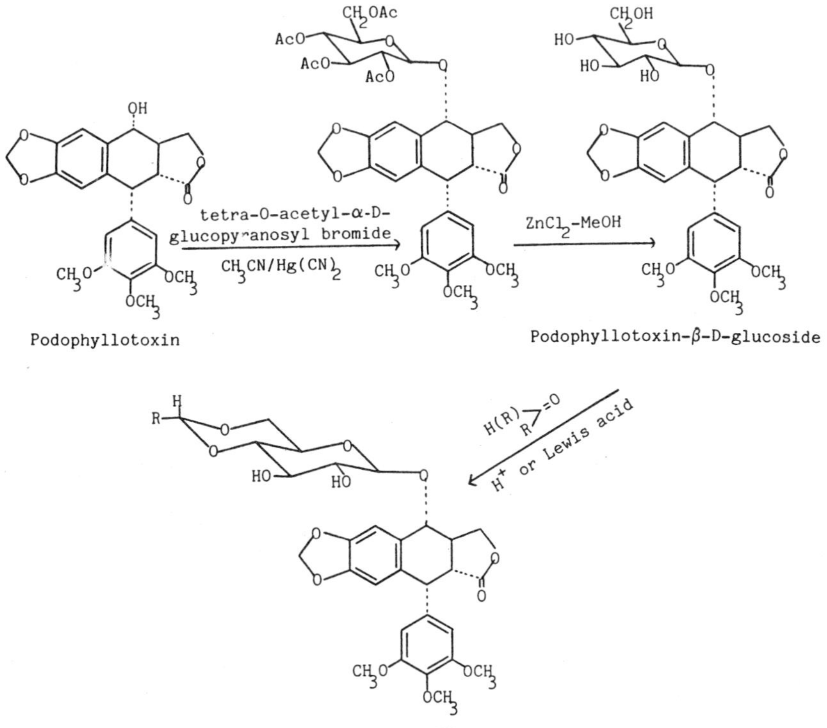

Podophyllotoxin

tetra-O-acetyl-α-D-glucopyranosyl bromide, $CH_3CN/Hg(CN)_2$

$ZnCl_2$-MeOH

Podophyllotoxin-β-D-glucoside

H(R)(R)C=O, H^+ or Lewis acid

Fig. 50

VP-16, 4'-demethylepipodophyllotoxin ethylidene β-D-glucoside, in contrast to other podophyllotoxins which are spindle poisons, appears to block entry of the cell into mitosis, acting during the late S and G_2 phases of the cell cycle. This compound is highly water insoluble. *In vitro* ED_{50} values against murine mastocytoma P-815 and HeLa cell are 0.046 μg/ml and 0.14

μg/ml, respectively. *In vivo* it showed inhibitory activity against sarcomas -37, -180, WM-256 carcinosarcoma, and P-815, P-1534, and L-1210 leukemias. In clinical trials (phase III), responses have been observed in patients with lymphoma, leukemia, brain tumor,

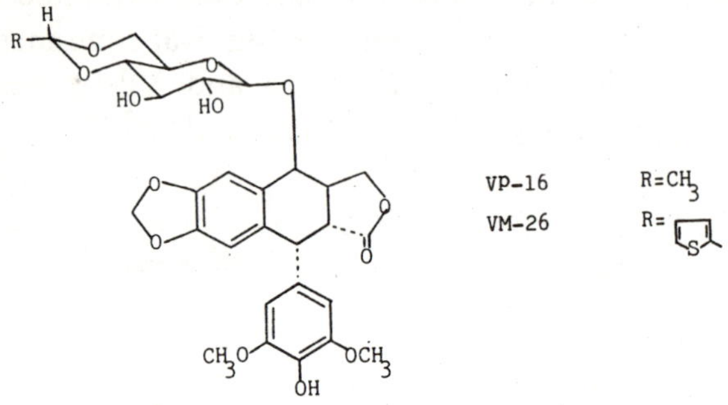

VP-16 R=CH_3
VM-26 R=

Fig. 51

lung cancer, breast cancer, bladder cancer, etc. Especially as a single agent, VP-16 is regarded to be the most active compound yet tested against small-cell bronchial carcinoma. Toxic effects include leukopenia, thrombocytopenia, alopecia, vomiting, and diarrhea; no long-term or cumulative toxicity has been reported, and all of these toxic effects are generally reversible when therapy is discontinued.[108]

VM-26, 4'-demethylepipodophyllotoxin thenylidene glucoside, in addition to producing mitotic arrest also inhibits entry of cells into mitosis, and leads to relatively rapid cell lysis. Pharmacological studies following intravenous administration of these agents have shown that VM-26 is excreted more slowly, but is metabolized faster than VP-16. In the initial clinical assessment, VM-26 has shown definite therapeutic activity in patients with Hodgkin's disease, bladder cancer, and presumably in CNS tumors. Limiting toxic manifestation appeared to be myelosuppression.[109]

In comparison with podophyllotoxins, epipodophyllotoxins seem to show lower inhibitory activity to microtubule assembly. The attachment of a glucoside moiety to position 4 of ring C of epipodophyllotoxin results in a reactant which has no effect on microbule assembly, the only remaining ability being to induce single-strand breaks in DNA; the breaks induced by VP-16 are reversible. It is the presence of the glucoside moiety that is responsible for this difference in action. However, the glucoside moiety itself is not necessary for the entirely different biological effect of VP-16, the presence of a 4'-hydroxy group at position 4' of ring E being regarded as important. Several nonglucoside podophyllotoxin derivatives which have a 4'-OH group at position 4' of ring E combine both the inhibitory actions on microtubule assembly and the ability to induce breaks in DNA. Obviously the podophyllotoxin ring system is an ideal structure for further modification in attempts to discover other antitumor agents.[110]

In order to block the conversion of transfused form to cis-fused form and resulting in biological deactivation of podophyllotoxin compounds, the lactone carbonyl group had been changed to methylene and other equivalent substituents. The defunctionalized podophyllotoxin derivatives, because they could not epimerize to the inner picropodophyllotoxin configuration, are expected to show enhanced biological properties. However, only the ring D cyclic ether derivatives retain considerable activity, indicating that although the lactone group of ring D is not required for activity, equivalent substitutions generally have less activity as the substitutions become more bulky, indicating strict requirements for the interaction of position 12 with tubulin.[111]

From the above structure-activity relationship studies, it can be concluded that the C and D rings of these compounds are involved in their interaction with tubulin, the activity of these compounds being specifically related to the configuration, size, and/or hydrophilic character of the C-4 position in the ring C and to the steric features of substituents at the 12th position of the D ring.

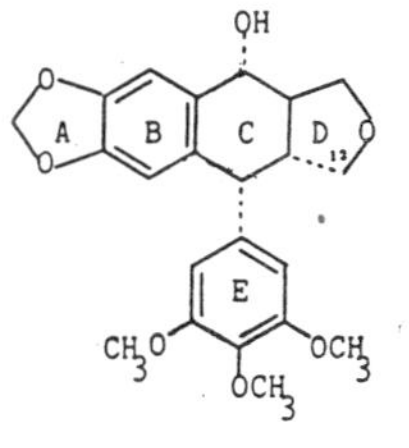

OH, A, B, C, D, 12, E, CH_3O, OCH_3, OCH_3

Podophyllotoxin cyclic ether (ID_{50} = 1.0 μM)

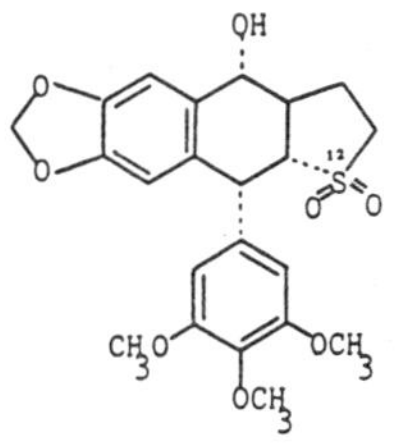

OH, 12, S, O, O, CH_3O, OCH_3, OCH_3

Podophyllotoxin cyclic sulfone (ID_{50} > 100 μM)

Fig. 52

7. Taxol

Taxol (V), a natural product derived from *Taxus brevifolia* (短葉紫杉) and other species of Taxaceae is a promising new antineoplastic agent. It has potent antileukemic and tumor-inhibiting properties. It is the first compound possessing the taxane ring that has demonstrated such activity.[112,113]

In L-1210, P-388, and P-1534 leukemia systems, taxol proves highly active. An inhibitor of WM-256 carcinosarcoma, it also showed considerable cytotoxicity in a KB assay (ED_{50} = 5.5 x 10^{-5} μg/ml). In addition, it was active in sarcoma-180 and Lewis lung cancers.

Taxol is an interesting drug in that it has a unique mechanism of action. Unlike other anticancer drugs, rather than inhibiting tubulin polymerization, it is an antimitotic agent and acts by promoting microtubule formation by decreasing the lag time for microtubule assembly and shifting the equilibrium in favor of the microtubule,[114] and decreasing the critical concentration of tubulin required for assembly, resulting in shorter microtubules. It markedly enhanced the tubulin polymerization, the microtubules formed in the presence of taxol usually being stable. This compound should soon be entering clinical trials.

Although taxol is an interesting and effective anticancer agent, it suffers from some disadvantages which might limit its usefulness. One major problem with the drug is its insolubility in water. Other problems are associated with its limited availability from natural sources and its potential instability. In an attempt to address these problems, a systematic investigation of structure-activity relationships in the field of the taxone diterpenes related to taxol has been undertaken.[115]

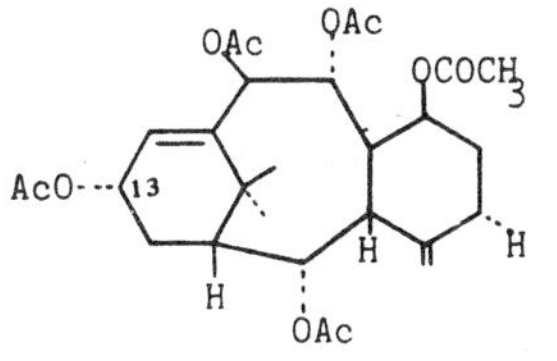

Fig. 53

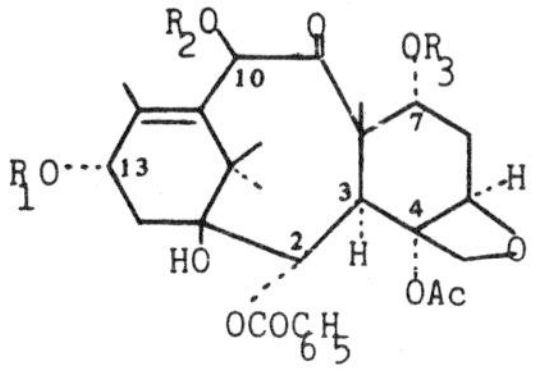

II $R_1 = R_2 = R_3 = H$
III $R_1 = COCH(OCOCH_3)CH(C_6H_5)NHCOC_6H_5$
$R_2 = R_3 = COCH_3$
IV $R_1 = COCH(OCOCH_3)CH(C_6H_5)NHCOC_6H_5$
$R_2 = H$ $R_3 = COCH_3$
V $R_1 = COCH(OH)CH(C_6H_5)NHCOC_6H_5$
$R_2 = COCH_3$ $R_3 = H$ (Taxol)

The results showed that none of the derivatives of taxol exhibited significant astrocyte reversal activity, and the esterification at C-13 appears to be essential for its activity. Some substituent changes, such as the loss of the acetyl group at C-10, apparently have little effect on the ability of taxol to assemble microtubules or to inhibit cell growth. However, acetylation at positions 7 and α-position on the C-13 side chain results in the abolition of activity. The two acetylated taxol derivatives (III and IV) showed significant activity in the KB cell culture assay,

Table 27. Biological Activity of Taxane Diterpenes[116]

Compound	Dose (μg/ml)	Astrocyte Reversal (duplicate assay)		ED_{50} (μg/ml) (in KB cell cul.)
I	100	6-13	16-33	28
II	100	16-30	16-30	1.0
III	100	16-30	16-30	0.03
IV	100	16-30	16-30	0.01
V	100	31-50	31-50	5.5×10^{-5}, 0.01

comparable to the activity shown by taxol itself. This suggests that the acetylated taxol may be converted intracellularly to taxol or other compounds with taxollike activity.[116]

8. Alkaloids

8.1 Vinca alkaloids

The discovery of vinblastine and vincristine, which play a significant role in the treatment of acute lymphocytic leukemia, aroused great interest in alkaloids in cancer treatment.[116] Vinblastine, a dimeric indole alkaloid isolated from *Catharanthus roseus* (L.) G. Don. (長春花 , *chang-chun-hua*), (Apocyanceae), can be converted into vincristine with higher antitumor activity and less toxicity by oxidation under reduced temperature.

The difference between the structure of vinblastine and vincristine is only in the substituent, a methyl or formyl group on the N_1 atom of the vindoline (lower) moiety. The "minor"

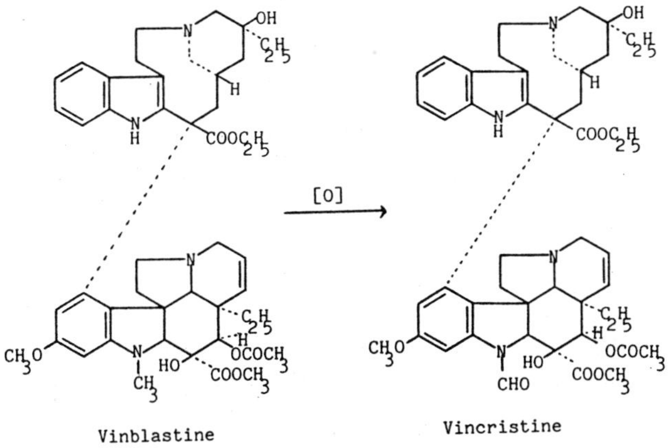

Fig. 54

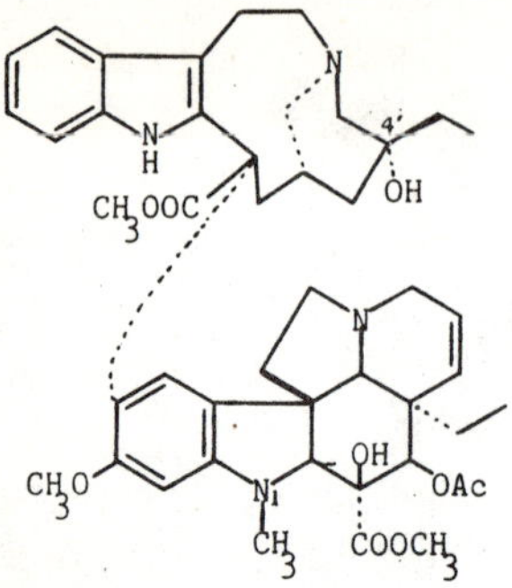

Leurosidine

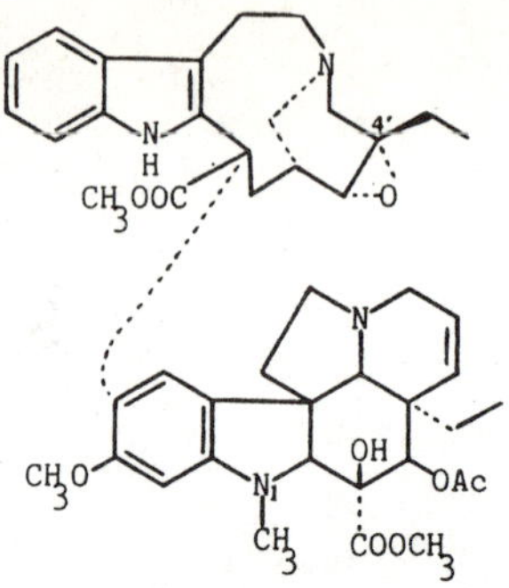

Leurosine

Fig. 55

changes in the vindoline moiety of vinblastine (VLB) do not cause loss of clinical activity, whereas such changes in the velbanamine (upper) moiety resulted in lower activity, such as the C-4' epimers leurosidine and leurosine. Thus VLB was favored as the parent alkaloid for modification, which resulted in a synthesis of vindensine and its derivatives.[118]

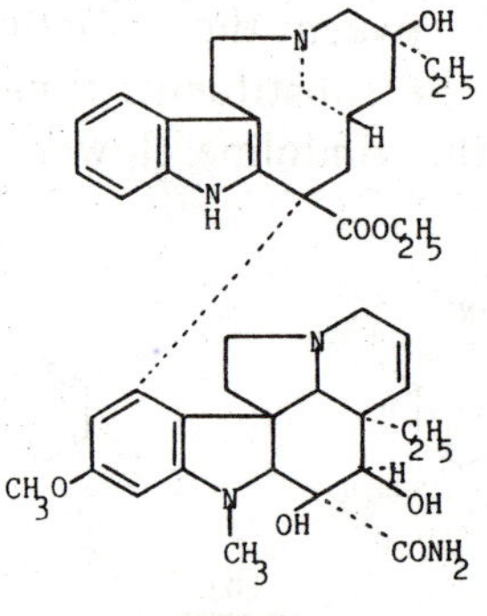

Vindensine

Fig. 56

Recently, vinblastine derivatives like vindensine were introduced into clinical use, because of their wider spectrum of antitumor activity in experimental systems and being less neurotoxic than vinblastine or vincristine.

Vinblastine and vincristine differ substantially in clinical utility and toxicity. Vinblastine is used clinically to treat solid tumors such as lymphoma and choriocarcinoma, while vincristine is primarily used for treatment of acute lymphocytic leukemia, especially acute leukemia in children. In this case, vincristine is often used in combination with 6-mercaptopurine and prednisone to produce induction remission and survival results not achieved in single-drug treatment. With regard to toxic effects vinblastine mainly restrains bone marrow, while vincristine adversly affects the peripheral nervous system.[118–122]

The biochemical mode of action is thought to involve the interaction of the vinca alkaloids with microtubular protein, which alters the tertiary structure of tubulin and hence the accessibility of the –SH group in tubulin.

The experimental antitumor spectrum of vindensine (VDS) resembles that of vincristine (VCR) rather than that of the parent VLB. Comparative acute toxicity studies of the VDS given I.V. to mice and rats yielded LD_{50} values between those of VLB and VCR in both species. Similarly, a phase II study of VDS in the treatment of breast carcinoma, malignant melanoma, and other tumors showed that VDS is a clinically active agent with a spectrum of toxicity between that of VCR and VLB.[121]

The functional changes associated with the conversion of VLB to VCR and VDS generate an additional hydrogen-bonding side in the vindoline moiety, and a decrease in lipophilicity in order of VLB > VDS > VCR.

Table 28. Uptake of H^3-vinca Alkaloids by Rat Lymphoma and L-5178Y Cells[a]

Alkaloid	Relative uptake*	P**	Relative tubulin* binding affinity
H^3-VLB	1	2.9	1
H^3-VCR	3.9	2.15	3.9
H^3-VDS	1	2.6	1.8

[a] From J. M. Cassady and J. D. Douros (edits), *Medicinal Chemistry, Anticancer Agents Based on Natural Product Models, A Series of Monograph,* Vol. 16, A Subsidiary of Harcourt Brace Jovanovich, Publishers, 1980.

*Relative to VLB = 1; **apparent partition coefficient in n-octanol/aqueous buffer solution at pH = 7.2.

According to a widely held notion, it is VLB, the more lipophilic member, that would be expected to penetrate more readily across nerve cell membranes and produce greater neurotoxicty. However contrary it seems, it has been shown that VCR has a higher uptake by nerve cells as well as by rat lymphoma and L-1578Y cells. At the same time, VCR is preferentially retained by these cells, resulting in high intracellular levels of VCR. In addition, determinations of the pharmacokinetics for the three drugs in patients indicate that VCR has the lowest and VLB the highest body clearance, with VDS in between. Thus differences in neurotoxicity and antitumor activity of VCR, VLB, and VDS may be attributed to differences in their actions at the cellular level and in their pharmacokinetics.[119,121]

Furthermore, a large number of VDS congeners (V-CONH-R) have been prepared from the azide (V-CON_3) and the appropriate amine. Generally in N-alkyl- and N-aralkyl-substituted vindesines, the introduction of larger alkyl substituents results in a loss of activity and increase in toxicity. N-β-hydroxyphenethyl

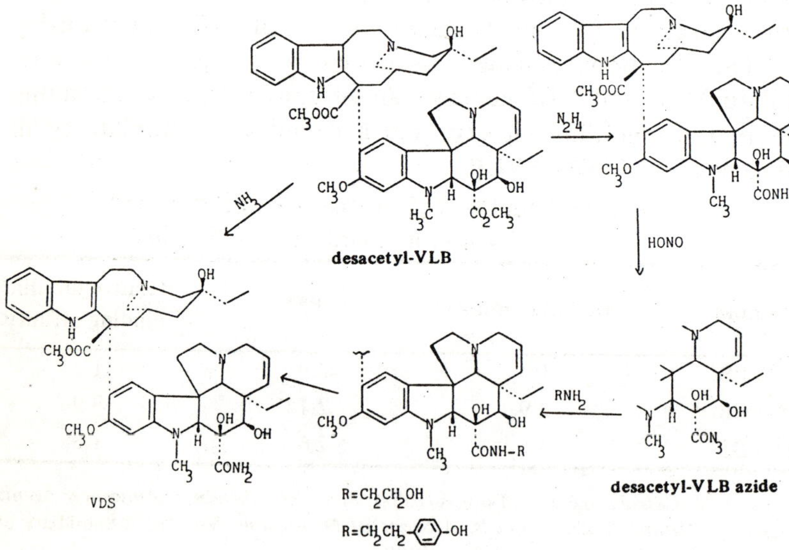

Fig. 57

VDS, though, is more active than VDS in the B-16 melanoma system.

In VDS congeners with N-alkyl groups bearing polar functions, the activity of N-β-hydroxyethyl VDS (V-$CONHCH_2CH_2OH$) equals or slightly surpasses that of VDS and even VCR, in terms of its therapeutic dose range.

8.2 Cephalotaxus alkaloids

Cephalotaxus (粗榧) is a genus of yewlike coniferous trees and shrubs consisting of seven species native to eastern Asia. This genus is the source of a unique group of alkaloids, the prototype of which is cephalotaxine.

Cephalotaxine (I) itself is inactive, while its four esters (II-V) exhibit various degrees of antitumor activity in the following experimental tumor systems: P-388 lymphocytic leukemia, L-1210 lymphoid leukemia, Lewis lung carcinoma, colon 38, and epidermoid carcinoma of the nasopharynx (KB cell culture). Harringtonine (II) was also found to be effective against L-615 leukemia, L-7212 leukemia, sarcoma-180, and Walker carcinosarcoma-256.[123-124]

Harringtonine (II) and homoharringtonine (III) show about the same activity in the P-388 leukemia system, and are both distinctly more active than deoxyharringtonine (IV) and isoharringtonine (V), indicating that insertion of an additional $-CH_2$

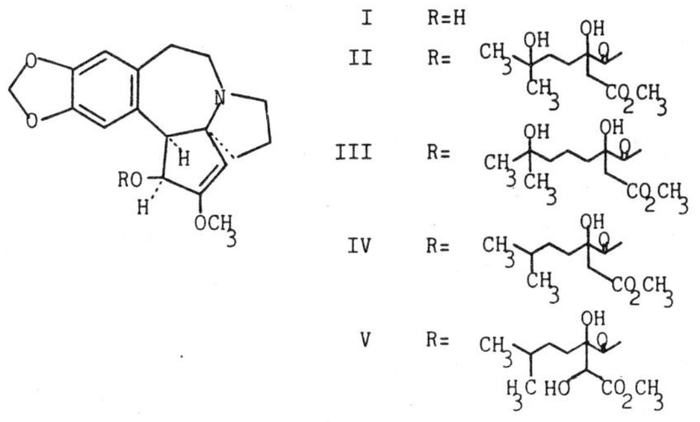

I R=H

II R=

III R=

IV R=

V R=

Fig. 58

group in the terminal portion of the acyl side chain of harringtonine has little effect on activity. On the other hand, removal of the OH group from the penultimate carbon of the acyl moiety (to give deoxyharringtonine) reduces activity by about half. Shifting this OH group to give isoharringtonine lowers P-388 activity by nearly one order of magnitude.[125]

Table 29. Antitumor Activity of Cephalotoxus Alkaloids Against P-388 Lymphocytic and L-1210 Lymphoid Leukemia in Mice

Compound	Dose (mg/kg)	T/C %	
		P-388	L-1210
I Cephalotaxine	110	–	107
II Harringtonine	1.0	405	135
	0.5	294	131
III Homoharringtonine	1.0	338	142
IV Deoxyharringtonine	2.0	180	–
	0.5	145	
V Isoharringtonine	7.5	272	126
	3.75	172	124

This information indicates that an ester linkage may be a structural requirement for antitumor activity, but it is insufficient in the absence of other features; indeed, the acid provided by hydrolysis of deoxyharringtonine and the corresponding dimethyl ester are inactive as well as natural (–)-cephalotaxine. Other esters of cephalotaxine, as well as cephalotaxine acetate, are also inactive.

Investigation has shown that these compounds inhibit protein synthesis in cell culture systems.

Clinical trials have demonstrated that harringtonine is effective in the treatment of lymphoma, Hodgkin's disease, choriocarcinoma, primary liver cancer, and leukemia. For instance, in treating 72 leukemia patients, 62 patients showed an objective response. Among them 24 achieved complete remission and 38 partial remission, the result being especially encouraging due to the fact that acute myelocytic leukemia had an overall remission rate of 86.1%.[126,127]

8.3 Camptothecin

Camptothecin was isolated from the wood, bark, and fruits of *Camptotheca acuminata* (喜樹) (Nyssaceae), [128] a tree native to China. Camptothecin possesses noteworthy activity in the mouse leukemia L-1210 system, with T/C values frequently in excess of 200. This is one of the few antineoplastic alkaloids that has shown consistently high activity in the resistant L-1210. All naturally occurring active principles in camptothecin series, including 10-hydroxycamptothecin, 10-methoxycamptothecin, and 9-methoxycamptothecin, with the exception of the sodium salt of camptothecin, show the same degree of broad-spectrum activity, with KB activity of the order 10^{-2} μg/ml. They also greatly inhibit the growth of solid tumors in animals.[118]

Table 30. Structures and Biological Activity of Camptothecin Alkaloids

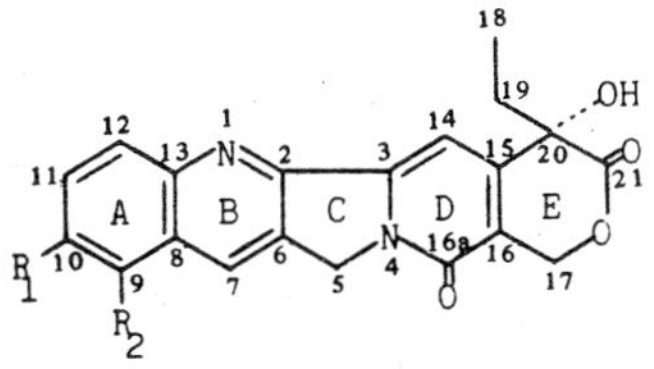

Compound	Structure	Biological Activity		
		PS T/C %	L-1210 T/C (mg/kg)	KB ED_{50} (μg/ml)
Camptothecin	$R_1=R_2=H$	250	230 (2.0)	2×10^{-2}
10-Hydroxycamptothecin	$R_1=OH$ $R_2=H$	268	230 (0.5-2.0)	2×10^{-2}
10-Methoxycamptothecin	$R_1=OMe$ $R_2=H$			
9-Methoxycamptothecin	$R_1=H$ $R_2=OMe$	217		

These ring A hydroxylated substances are found only as trace constituents along with the major product, campthothecin. They may be produced as a result of further plant metabolism.

The structural characteristics of camptothecin are the presence of a conjugated A, B, C, D ring system and an α-hydroxy-lactone moiety ring E in its molecule.

(1) Importance of the α-hydroxy-lactone ring

After acetylation of the α-hydroxy group or replacement of this group by chlorine and hydrogen, all the resultant C-20 acetate (I), chloro analogues (II), and corresponding deoxy analogues (III) are inactive in L-1210 and P-388 leukemia tests. Reduction of the lactone ring resulted in the lactol (IV) having greatly reduced activity.

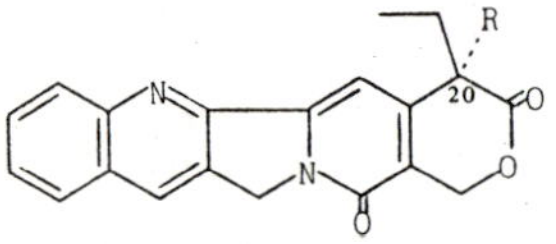

(I) R=OAc
(II) R=Cl
(III) R=H

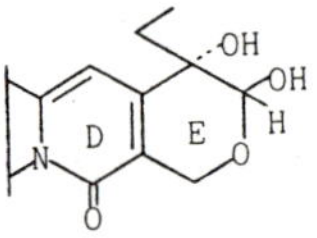

(IV) Lactol analogue

Fig. 59

On the other hand, as shown in Figure 60, some N-alkyl amide analogues (V-VII), as well as the sodium salt of camptothecin (VIII) have *in vivo* antitumor activity. Although they lack the lactone ring, the α-hydroxy lactone moiety can be regenerated by recyclization in dilute acid. However, compound (IX) which has a carbon-nitrogen bond at C-17 cannot be hydrolyzed and recycled to regenerate the α-hydroxy lactone

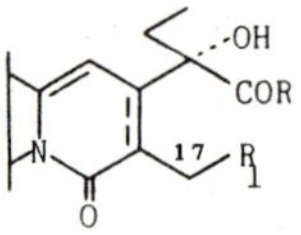

(V) R=HNMe R_1=OH
(VI) R=HNCHMe$_2$ R_1=OH
(VII) R=HNCHMe$_2$ R_1=OAc
(VIII) R=ONa R_1=OH
(IX) R=HNCHMe$_2$ R_1=-N

Fig. 60

ring; this compound proves completely inactive in several *in vivo* leukemia systems.[11]

These findings suggest that the intact α-hydroxy lactone ring E is absolutely required for antitumor activity of camptothecin.

(2) Substitution of A ring[11]

Introduction of certain substituents in ring A at the 9, 10, and 12 positions may result in increased activity. 10-Hydroxycamptothecin is the most active compound in the camptothecin series, having both a significantly higher T/C and a lower optimal dose than other compounds in the series tested so far. Since sodium salt of camptothecin has been shown to be clinically inactive, it was hoped that the preparation of a water soluble salt from a ring A derivative would give the desirable combination of water solubility and the intact α-hydroxy lactone ring. (Figure 61)

However, the two water soluble ethers (X) and (XI) are inactive; the electrostatic interaction between negative charge of the carboxylate anion of (X) and that of the phosphate group of DNA may prevent DNA binding. For compound (XI), this

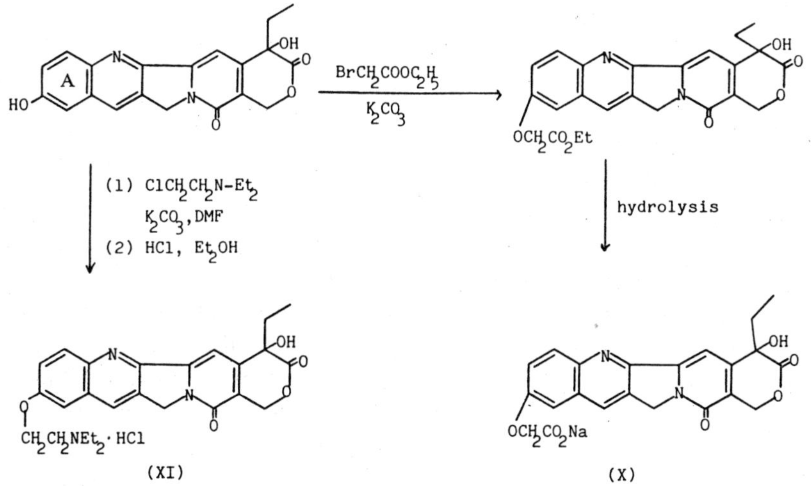

HO, A, N, OH, O

$BrCH_2COOC_2H_5$

K_2CO_3

OCH_2CO_2Et

(1) $ClCH_2CH_2N\text{-}Et_2$

K_2CO_3, DMF

(2) HCl, Et_2OH

hydrolysis

$CH_2CH_2NEt_2 \cdot HCl$

(XI)

OCH_2CO_2Na

(X)

Fig. 61

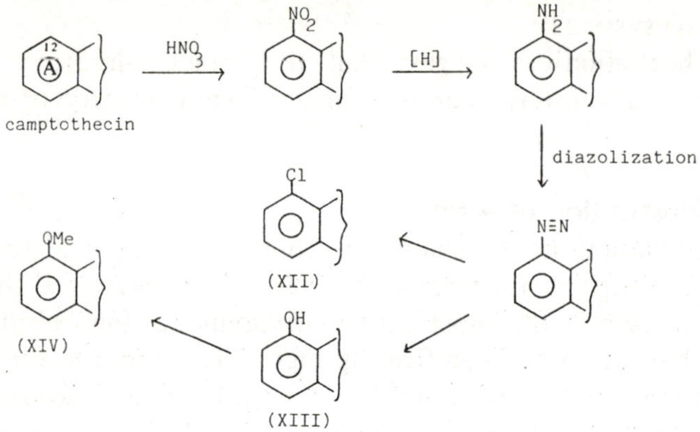

camptothecin

HNO$_3$

[H]

diazolization

(XII)

(XIII)

(XIV)

Fig. 62

may be due to steric or electronic interference of the diethylaminoethoxy moiety.

Among 12-substituted analogues (Figure 62), the 12-chloro analogue (XII) was reported to be very active in L-615 leukemia screening. Semisynthetic compounds like 12-hydroxy (XIII) and 12-methoxy (XIV) analogues were more active against Ehrlich ascites carcinoma.

3) Number of rings

It has been shown that the simple monocyclic ring E, bicyclic ring DE, and tricyclic ring CDE analogues (XV-XIX) containing the α-hydroxy lactone moiety prove completely inactive in the *in vivo* leukemia systems, in KB cytotoxicity, in inhibition of RNA synthesis, and in depolymerization of DNA.[11] On the basis of molecular orbital analysis, a tetracyclic system containing BCDE rings was proposed to be the minimum size structure for biological activity in the camptothecin series.

The pentacyclic analogue DL-camptothecin was active but less potent than camptothecin, indicating that the S-configuration at C-20 is required for maximal antitumor activity. Thus it was reasonable that DL-10-hydroxy-camptothecin would be one-half as potent as the corresponding natural alkaloid.

Other pentacyclic analogues such as 12-azacamptothecin and thiophene analogue were less active and much less potent

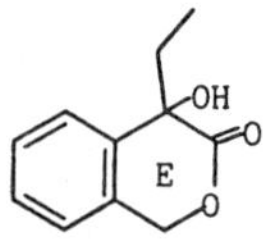

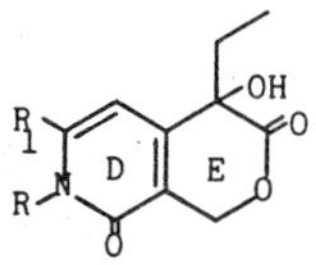

(XV) R=H, R_1=Me
(XVI) R=n-C_4H_9, R_1=Me
(XVII) R=β-naphthylmethyl R_1=H

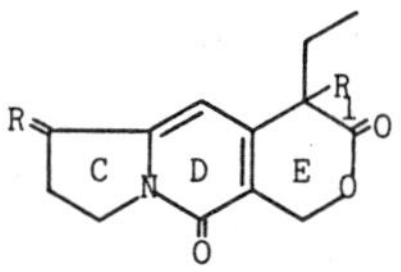

(XVIII) R=H, R_1=OH
(XIX) R=O, R_1=H

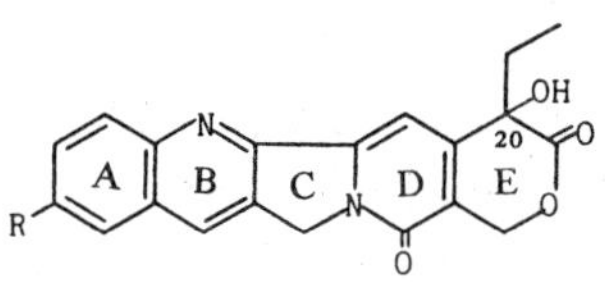

DL-camptothecin R=H
DL-10-hydroxycamptothecin R=OH
DL-10-methoxycamptothecin R=OMe

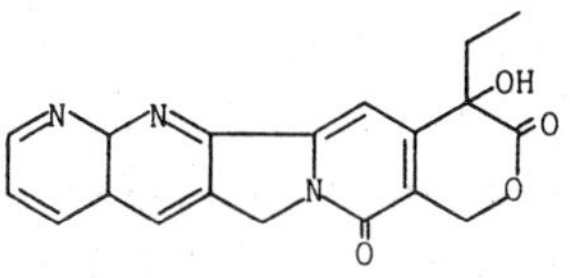

12-Aza analogue

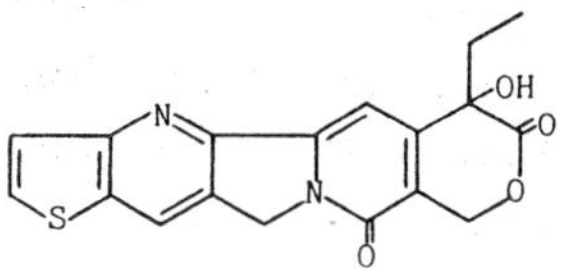

Thiophene analogue

Fig. 63

than DL-camptothecin. This may be due to electronic interference of pyridine and the thiophene ring with intercalation between the two base pairs of DNA.

The DL-hexacyclic analogue (XX) was found to have the same order of activity as camptothecin but was about one-half as potent in the P-388 leukemia system.

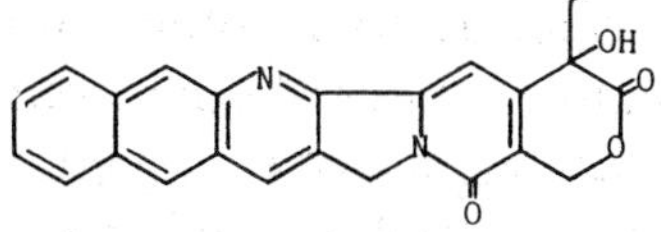

(XX)

Fig. 64

In summary, camptothecin is an inhibitor of DNA and causes conversion of cellular DNA to lower molecular weight species. This process seems to bc more sensitive to alterations in ring E, but only compounds with an -OH group adjacent to the carbonyl are active in degradation of DNA, although inhibition of RNA synthesis seems to be a general property of camptothecin and all analogues which have the conjugated A, B, C, D ring system. Thus, the activity of camptothecin might be due to two factors: (a) a flat, planar structure which would be required for binding with nucleic acids by intercalation; (b) the α-hydroxy lactone moiety must be available.

In addition to the camptothecin series, other naturally occurring compounds possessing a similar conjugate planar structure to that of camptothecin and antitumor activity include: acronycine,[129,130] tylocrebrine,[131,132] ellipticine, indirubin, some podophyllotoxines, and antitumor antibiotics such as pluramycin, kidamycin, and so on. Some of these compounds were found to intercalate with DNA and to be inhibitors of RNA and DNA synthesis.

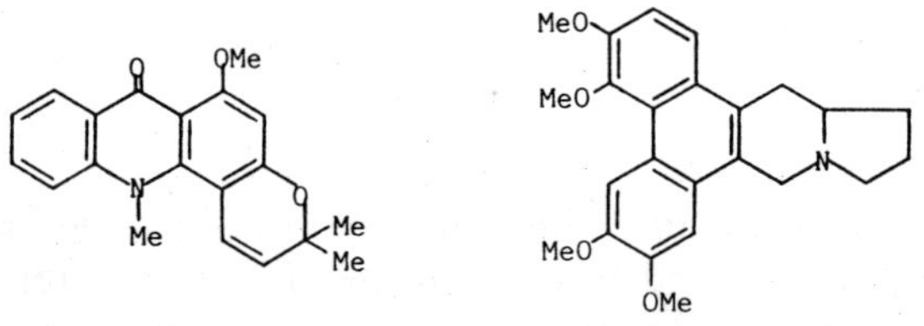

Acronycine

Tylocrebrine

Fig. 65

Among a wide variety of polycyclic molecules known to bind DNA by intercalation, actinomycin and daunomycin have essential side chains, whereas some others do not and may be considered to be "simple" intercalating agents. These are distinguished by a tendency for lower binding strength, faster kinetics of reaction and dissociation, and less specificity for binding to helical DNA. Ellipticine was found to resemble the simple intercalators.[133]

8.4 Ellipticine alkaloids

Ellipticine and analogues are alkaloids isolated from the Australian plant *Ochrosia moorei* (Apocyanceae). Another plant of the same genus, *Ochrosia borbonica* (旁波玫瑰樹), has been introduced in Yunnan province in China.

Ellipticines have been shown to have significant antitumor activities against several experimental tumors, including L-1210, P-388, and sarcoma-180. Among these alkaloids, 9-OH-ellipticine elicits high antitumor activity in L-1210 mouse leukemia at low doses, whereas high doses have less activity than expected because of a leveling off of the antitumor dose-activity relationship. A few cell lines were resistant to the treatment.[134–136]

The study of 16 homologues of ellipticine indicated that 5-methyl-, 6-methyl-, 1,5-dimethyl-, 5,11-dimethyl-, 9-methoxyl-5,11-dimethyl-, and 9-methoxyl-5,6,11-trimethyl-ellipticinum all have antitumor activity, but 3-methyl-, 9-methyl-, 5,7,10,11-

Table 31. Structure and Cytotoxicity of Some Ellipticine Derivatives

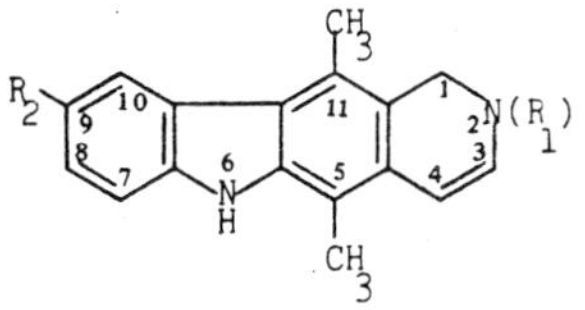

CH_3 R_2 10   9   8   7   6   N   H   11   5   1   2   N(R_1)   3   4 CH_3

Compound	Structure R_1	R_2	ED_{50} for DC-3F (M)*	ED_{50} Ratio (DC-3F/9-OH-E 0.3: DC-3F)**
Ellipticine	–	H $\Delta^{1,2}$	1.6×10^{-7}	4
9-OH-ellipticine	–	OH $\Delta^{1,2}$	3.0×10^{-7}	10
9-CH_3O-ellipticine	–	CH_3O $\Delta^{1,2}$	3.0×10^{-7}	4
2-CH_3-ellipticinum	CH_3	H	2.4×10^{-6}	10
2-CH_3-9-OH-ellipticinum	CH_3	OH	1.2×10^{-6}	16
2-CH_3-9-CH_3COO-ellipticinum	CH_3	CH_3COO	1.7×10^{-6}	21

*The parental line of Chinese hamster lung cells

**The DC-3F/9-OH-E 0.3 subline is Chinese hamster lung cells resistant to ellipticine derivatives.

tetramethyl-, and 9-bromo-ellipticinum are inactive. In human oncology, 9-methoxy-ellipticine has been used successfully in the treatment of acute myeloblastic leukemia. The therapeutic value of 9-hydroxy-2-methyl-ellipticinum in advanced cancer, especially in breast cancer, has been reported. It is recently being used in phase II and phase III trials in several countries. The phase II studies have demonstrated that it has some activities in thyroid and kidney carcinomas, soft tissue sarcomas, and advanced breast cancer.[136]

The main characteristic of 9-hydroxy-2-methyl ellipticinum is its lack of marrow toxicity. The major and most unpleasant side effect was an inhibition of salivary secretion, which causes other complications such as tongue mycosis, anorexia, and asthenia. Other side effects were nausea with or without vomiting, xerostoma, stomatitis, and neurologic toxicity. It has been shown that this compound rapidly accumulates in the gastrointestinal walls and salivary and thyroid glands, which suggests that there may be a correlation between the noted uptake and the response observed in thyroid cancer and the side effect of dryness of mouth.

The mechanism of action of ellipticine alkaloids is the inhibition of DNA, RNA, and protein synthesis. These alkaloids consist of planar heterocyclic ring systems. It is uncharged at neutral pH but acquires a positive charge under mildly acid conditions (pK_a of 5.8). This type of structure suggests intercalation between base pairs of helical nucleic acids as a possible mode of action. Ellipticine has been observed to interact with DNA and increases its melting point. *In vivo,* it has also been shown to induce single-strand breaks in protein-associated DNA. The 9-methoxy derivative of ellipticine has been reported to produce viscosity changes indicative of intercalation.[134]

8.5 Benzophenanthridine alkaloids

Benzophenanthridine alkaloids possess interesting biological and pharmacological properties. Among these, nitidine chloride and 6-methoxy-5,6-dihydronitidine isolated from *Zanthoxylum*

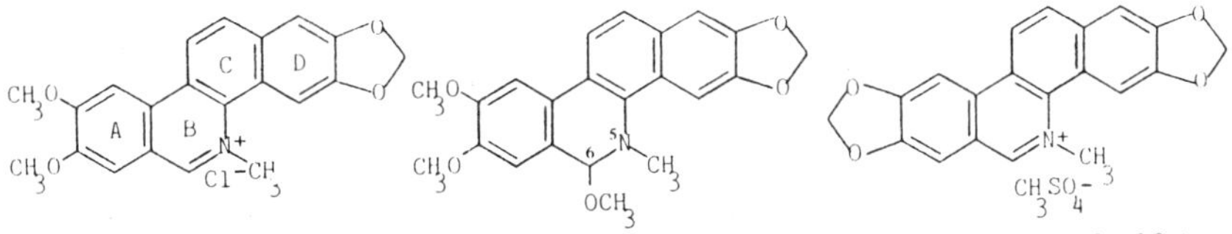

Nitidine chloride   6-Methoxy-5,6-dihydronitidine   Allonitidine methylsulfate

Fig. 66

nitidum (兩面針 , *liang menchen*) (Rutaceae) were found to be highly cytotoxic.[137–139] They exhibited antileukemic activity in both leukemic L-1210 and P-388 systems in mice and inhibited Lewis lung carcinoma. Synthetic 6-methoxy-5,6-dihydronitidine and allonitidine also showed antileukemic activity. Nitidine chloride has been chosen for preclinical pharmacologic and toxicologic evaluation.

It has been reported that these alkaloids possess inhibitory activity against reverse transcriptase of RNA tumor viruses. The mechanism of action is interaction with adenine-thymine (A:T) template primers and stopping DNA synthesis at the initiation of the polymerization processes. Thus they could be promising prophylactic agents in cancer prevention.[139]

In order to decrease the cytotoxic action and to increase the inhibitory activity of these alkaloids against leukemia, a number of synthetic programs with the aim of potentiating their activity has been initiated, but so far no compound has been found with activity higher than that of nitidine chloride. Any modification of the D-ring decreases the activity. Modification of ring A has been suggested.[140–142]

Closely related to the benzophenanthridines are the berberine alkaloids. Berberine showed only *in vitro* activity in the Ehrlich ascites test system in the dose range of 2.5-7.5 mg/kg/day, while berberoline and thiophosphamide derivatives of berberine have exhibited antitumor activity.[80]

Tetrandrine, the main alkaloid isolated from the Chinese drug *Stephania tetrandra* (漢防己 , *han-fang-chi*), showed enough activity in the Walker-256 intramuscular carcinoma test system to be considered for preclinical toxicologic evaluation.

This alkaloid is also contained in the Chinese drugs *Stephania*

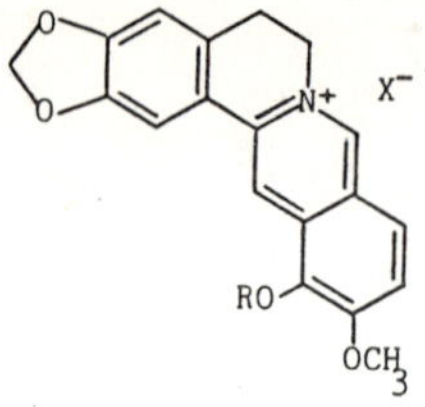

Berberine R=CH_3
Berberoline R=H

Fig. 67

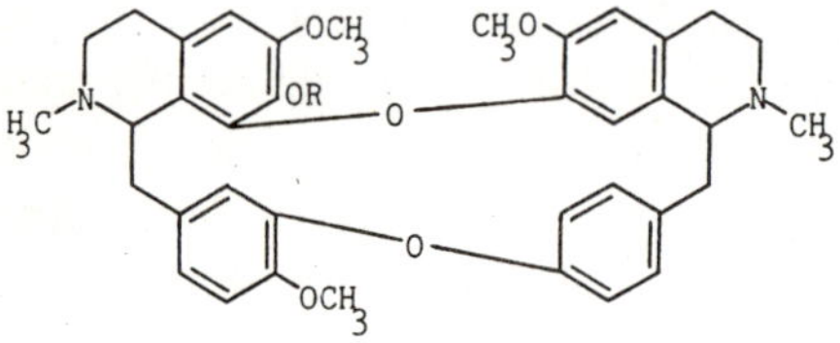

Tetrandrine R=CH_3
Fangchinoline R=H

Fig. 68

japonica Miers (千金藤, *ch'ien-chin t'eng*) and *Cocculus laurifollus* DC. (衡州烏藥, *henzhou wuyao*) (Menispermaceae.)[80]

8.6 Pyrrolizidine alkaloids – monocrotaline and indicine-N-oxide

Pyrrolizidine alkaloids are generally found in *Crotalaria* and the *Senecio* genera of Compositae, and the subfamilies of Heliotropioideae and Boraginoideae of Boraginaceae. Monocrotaline isolated from *Crotalaria sessiliflora* L. (農吉利, *nung-chili*) has been used effectively for the treatment of skin cancer.

Monocrotaline and many other pyrrolizidine alkaloids, such as senecionine, indicine-N-oxide, and heliotrine are derived from retronecine or its isomer, heliotridine, the difference being only in the ester moiety.

Culvenor[143] examined eighteen pyrrolizidine alkaloids and several derivatives for tumor inhibitory properties and found 10 of 23 compounds tested active at significant levels against one or more tumor systems (Table 32). The tumors most frequently inhibited are Walker-256 intramuscular (WM) and adenocarcinoma-755 (CA). Among the monocrotaline type, monocrotaline and spectabiline were observed to possess a high level of activity against adenocarcinoma-755 (CA), the highest degree of inhibition being achieved (95%) at a dose of 90 mg/kg. It was

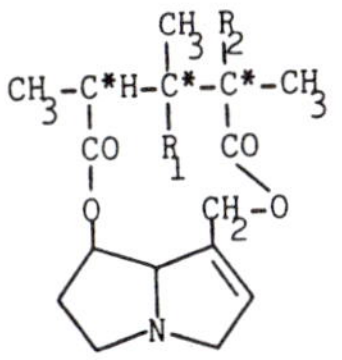

Monocrotaline R_1=OH R_2=OH
Fulvine, crispatine R_1=OH, R_2=OH
Spectabiline R_1=OCOCH$_3$, R_2=OH
Monocrotaline R_1R_2= -OCH(CH$_3$)O-

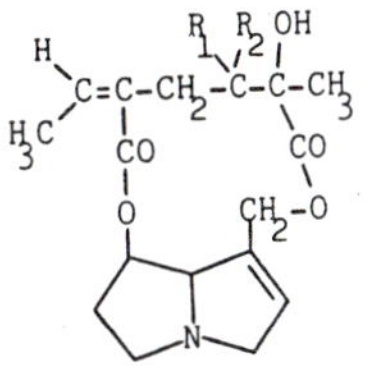

Senecionine R_1=H, R_2=CH$_3$
Seneciphylline R_1R_2=-CH$_2$-

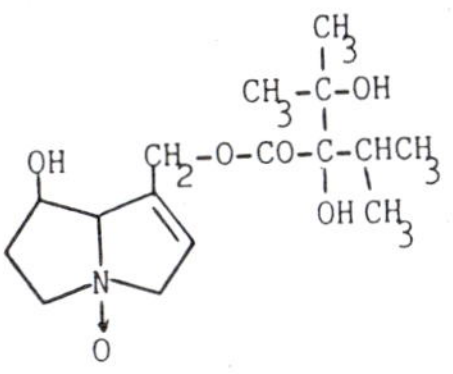

Indicine-N-oxide

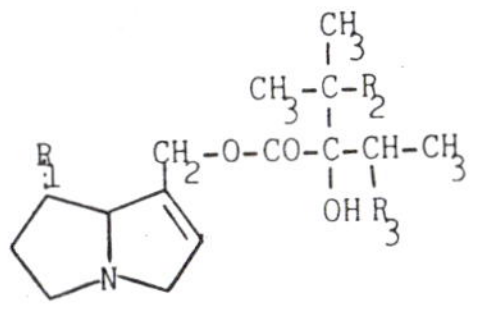

Heliotrine R_1=OH, R_2=H, R_3=OCH$_3$
Echinatine R_1=OH, R_2=H, R_3=OH

Fig. 69

also reported to be active against WM, plasmacytoma and sarcoma-180. The alkaloids of the senecionine type with a 12-member cyclic diester have proved to be highly active against WM at low dose levels, but they also prove highly toxic to the host. Of the bases of the heliotrine type, heliotrine and indicine N-oxide are strongly active against WM. Significant activity was observed with indicine N-oxide in WM, L-1210, P-388, P-1535 leukemia, and melanoma B-16 tumor systems.[144] On the basis of these results, indicine N-oxide was selected for human clinical trials by the CCNSC. The clinical evaluation of indicine N-oxide is clearly at an early stage. The drug has not only been active in usually resistant solid tumors (colon carcinoma and malignant melanoma), but has also shown activity in patients with refractory leukemia.[145]

In vivo, the pyrrolizidine alkaloid is metabolized by the liver microsome to dehydropyrrolizidine derivatives, which as alkylating agents are thought to be the type responsible for the antitumor activity as well as the acute toxic effects of the alkaloids,[146–149] as shown in Figure 70.

Table 32. Antitumor Screen* of Pyrrolizidine Alkaloids

Alkaloids	CA	LE	SA	WM	WA	KB	Toxicity**
monocrotaline	+	–	+	+	–	–	+
spectabiline	+	–		+	+	–	
fulvine	+	–	–	+	+	–	++
crispatine	+	–	–	–	–	–	++
heliotrine	+		+	+	–	–	+
lasiocarpine		–	+	+	+	–	++
europine					–	–	±
echinatine	–	–			–	–	±
supinine	+	–	–	–	–	–	±
heleurine	–	–	–	–	–	–	±
senecionine	–	–	–	+	–	–	++
seneciphylline	–	–	–	–	–	–	
monocrotaline N-oxide	–	–					
sarracine	–	–	–	–			
heliotrine N-oxide	–	–	–	+		+	
indicine N-oxide		+		+			–
retronecine HCl		–	–				–
1-methoxymethyl 1-7β-hydroxy-1,2-hydro-pyrrolizidine						–	
1-methylene-pyrrolizidine		–		–	–		–
1-chloromethyl-7α-hydroxy-1,2-dehydro-pyrrolizidine	+		+			–	++

* CA: adenocarcinoma-755; LE: lymphoid leukemia L-1210; SA: sarcoma-180; WM: Walker-256 intramuscular; WA: Walker-256 subcutaneous; KB: cell culture.

** The sign "+" and the sign "–" symbolize comparative hepatotoxicity from reference 143.

It has been shown that a high ratio between the tertiary amine bases and their N-oxides in the plant increases the toxicity of pyrrolizidine alkaloid-containing plants, and that high hepatotoxicity correlates with high lipid solubility and low basicity. The active pyrrolizidine alkaloids are all of the allylic ester type which have a potential for alkylation. The ester of the saturated pyrrolizidine aminoalcohols lacking the $C_{1,2}$-double bond has neither antitumor activity nor hepatotoxicity, just like their free aminoalcohols. Their antitumor activity seems quite definitely to be associated with the same functional region in the molecule as hepatotoxicity. But, indicine N-oxide, which has a favorable ratio of antitumor activity to toxicity, appears to be unique among the pyrrolizidine alkaloids. It is possible that its antitumor effects may not be mediated through the formation of indicine and dehydroindicine.

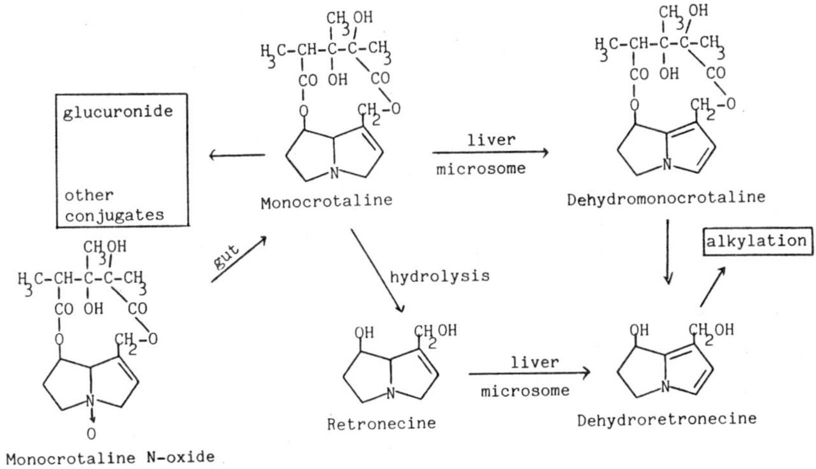

Fig. 70

Because of the potential hepatotoxicity and carcinogenicity of pyrrolizidine alkaloids and their metabolite dehydrorectonecine, further research is needed before they can be put to wide use.

9. Others

9.1 Maytansinoides

Table 33. Structure and Antitumor Activity of Maytansinoides

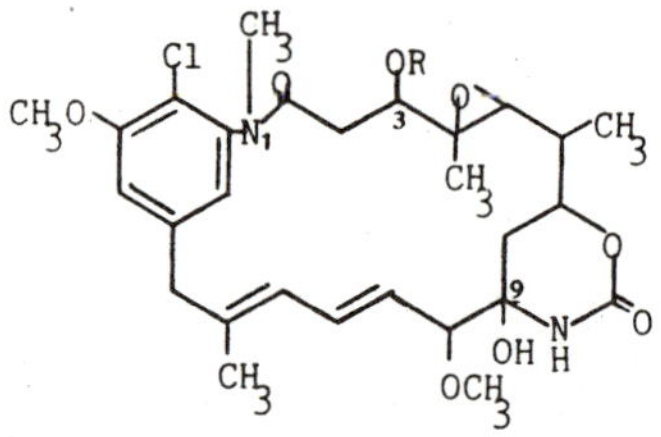

Compound	Structure	Antitumor Activity P-388 T/C (μg/kg)	KB Cell ED_{50} (μg/ml)
Maytansine	R = COCHMe (NMeCOMe)	220 (25)	6.1×10^{-6}
Maytanvalin	R = $COCHMeNMeCOCH_2(Me)_2$	187 (12.5)	2.3×10^{-7}
Maysine	C_3 = O	80 (50)	2.5×10^{-2}
Maytansinol	R = H	–	–
Normaysine	N_1 - H R = H	115 (3.1)	1.9×10^{-2}

Maytansine, isolated from *Maytanus oratus, M. serrata, M. buchananii,* and *M. hookeri* (美登木) (Celastraceae) found in the south of Yunnan province of China, was once regarded as a very promising anticancer agent because of its very strong inhibitory action on P-388 in mice at μg/kg dose range, with an ED_{50} of 10^{-4} - 10^{-5} μg/ml to KB cells. It is also very effective against S-180, Lewis lung cancer, L-1210, and WM-256.[152]

A maytansinoide is regarded as benzenic ansamycin in which the aromatic moiety is joined at two nonadjacent positions by an aliphatic ansa chain. The large substituent at C-3 and the hydroxyl group at C-9 are hydrophilic regions of the molecule, in contrast to the rest of the molecule which is hydrophobic. Compounds which lack the C-3 ester are less active than those with the ester. Conversion of C-9 alcohol of the carbinalamide to an ester is accompanied by a marked decrease in antileukemic activity and cytotoxicity against KB cells.

It has been established that maytansine mitosis in sea urchin eggs and L-1210 leukemia cells is by interaction with the microtubule system of the cells. Like the vinca alkaloids, vincristine and vinblastine, maytansine binds to tubulin at the same site and prevents its polymerization to microtubules. In this process, the C-3 ester linkage appears to be important in the tubulin-maytansinoide interaction, and the presence of the free C-9 –OH of the carbinolamide appears to aid the ability of maytansinoides to inhibit tubulin polymerization, suggesting that the compound may interact with tubulin at two sites. Of course, esterification of the C-3 –OH group may also facilitate drug transport into the cells.

Phase I clinical studies of maytansine have been conducted using the dose range of 0.01 to 0.8 mg/m^2/day with a total dose of 2.5 mg, in the treatment of breast cancer, ovarian cancer, non-Hodgkin's lymphoma, melanoma, and head and neck cancer. Some therapeutic benefits have been obtained.[153-155] Frequently encountered toxic effects are nausea, vomiting, diarrhea, stomatitis, and alopecia. It is interesting that a lack of cross-resistance between maytansine and vincristine exists. They were found to differ in the manner in which they inhibit microtubule assembly.[156]

However, the activity of the compound has been disappointing, as no objective responses to maytansine were reported in several phase II trials.[157-159]

Many homologous antileukemic ansa macrolides have been isolated from several *Maytanus* and *Putterlickia* species (Celastraceae), from *Colubrina texensis* (Rhamnaceae), and more recently from fermentation broths of *Nocardio* species. Among them, normaytansine was found to have significant *in vivo* activity against P-388 lymphocytic leukemia in mice at doses comparable to maytansine (T/C 181 at 100 μg/kg) and *in vitro* activity against the KB cell culture (ED_{50} = 10^{-3} μg/ml).[160]

9.2 Indirubin

Indigo (*ging dai*), a product derived from the leaves of *Baphicacanthus cusis* (馬藍 , *ma-lan*), has been revealed to be effective against leukemic L-7212 in mice. Indirubin was identified as the active antitumor principle. It showed various inhibitory activities against Walker carcinoma in rats and Lewis lung cancer in mice, as well as mammary cancer Ca-615 and L-7212 in mice. The clinical trial showed that of 314 patients with chronic myelocytic leukemia, 82 achieved complete remission, 38 partial remission, and 87 beneficial effects. The total effective rate was 87.3%. It has been shown to have a therapeutic effect similar to myleran (1,4-butanediol dimethanesulfonate) in treatment of chronic myelocytic leukemia, and neither serious side effects nor inhibition of bone marrow was observed.[11]

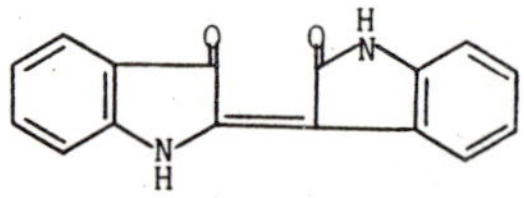

Indirubin

Fig. 71

Other Chinese drugs with anticancer activities are listed in Table 34.

Table 34. Chinese Drugs and Related Plants Used to Treat Cancer

Plants	Active Principle	Anticancer Activity	Reference
Acanthaceae			
Acanthus ilicifolius 老鼠簕			2
Baphicacanthus cusis 馬藍	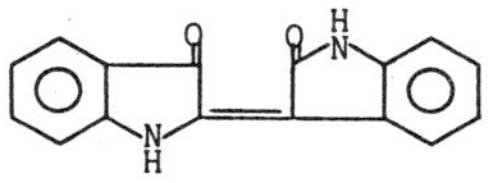 Indirubin	effective against leukemic L-7212 in mice, inhibits WM-256, Lewis lung cancer and mammary cancer Ca-615. Clinical application: indirubin has a similar therapeutic effect to myleran in treatment of chronic myelocytic leukemia.	11
Justicia procumbens 爵床草			2
J. flava	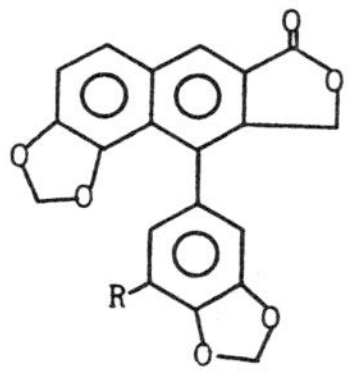 Helioxanthin R=H Justicinol R=OH 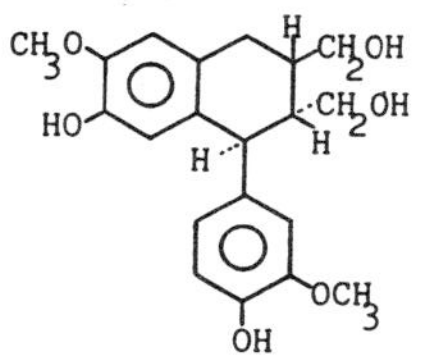 Isolariciresinol	against P-388	162
Aceraceae			
Acer negundo 梣葉槭		inhibits WM-256	163

Chinese Drugs and Related Plants Used to Treat Cancer

Plants	Active Principle	Anticancer Activity	Reference
Actinidiaceae *Actinidia chinensis* 藤梨根	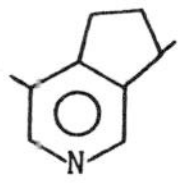 Actinidia alkaloids		2
Agavaceae *Agave schottii* 龍舌蘭	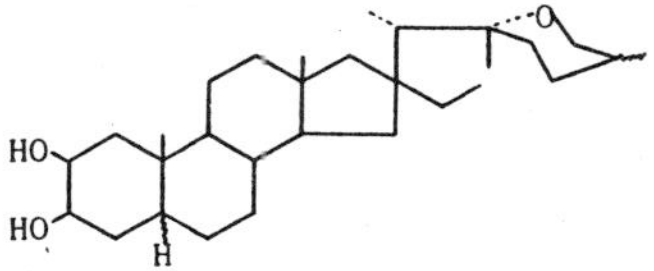 Gitogenin	inhibits WM-256	164
Amaryllidaceae *Narcissus tazetta* L. var. *chinensis* Roemer 中國水仙	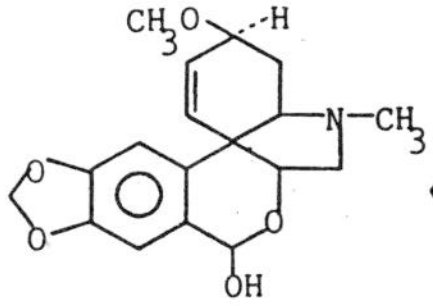 Pretazettine 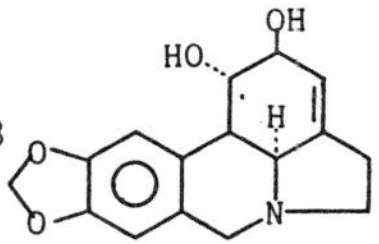 Lycorine	inhibits animal tumors	165, 166

Plants	Active Principle	Anticancer Activity	Reference
Apocynaceae			
Catharanthus roseus 長春花	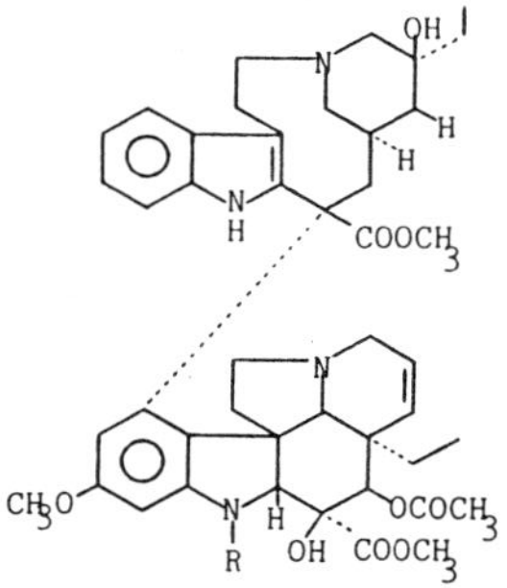 Vinblastine $R=CH_3$ Vincristine $R=CHO$	P-1534, L-1210, Akr-leukemia, WM-256, IRC 741/1398 leukemia, S-180, EA uses: vinblastine: solid tumor such as Hodgkin's disease and other lymphoma vincristine: acute lymphocytic leukemia	111, 118, 119
Aquifoliaceae			
Ilex cornuta 枸骨			2
Araceae			
Amorphophallus konjac 蛇六谷			2
Pinellia pedatisecta 掌葉半夏		folklore remedy for tumors	4

Chinese Drugs and Related Plants Used to Treat Cancer

Plants	Active Principle	Anticancer Activity	Reference
Araliaceae			
Panax ginseng 人參	total saponins		236
Aristolochiaceae			
Atractylodes macrocephala 白朮	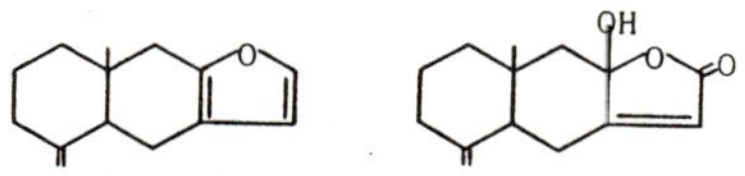 Atractylon (I) Butenolide (II)	showed activity against esophageal cancer Ca-109, *in vitro*	11
Ervatamia divaricata 狗牙花			2
E. dichotoma (Roxb.) Blatter		the alkaloids isolated from petroleum ether extract showed antitumor activity	167
E. heyneama	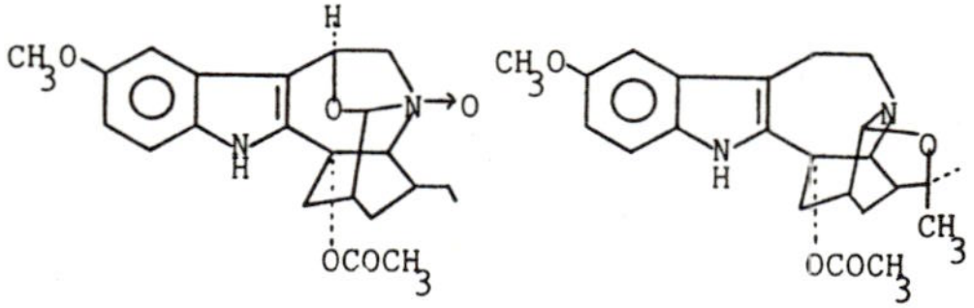 10-methoxyeglandine-N-oxide (-)-heyneatine	against P-388, ED_{50} = 1.6 and 3.8 μg/ml, respectively	5

Chinese Drugs and Related Plants Used to Treat Cancer

Plants	Active Principle	Anticancer Activity	Reference
Trachelospermum jasminoides 絡石藤	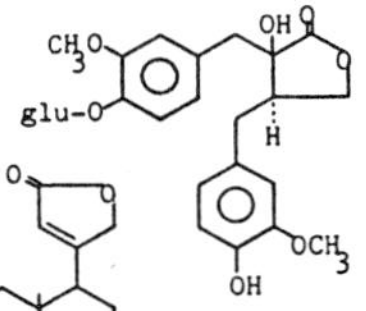 Nortracheloside		2
T. asiaticum 日本絡石			167
Thevetia ahouia 黃花夾竹桃	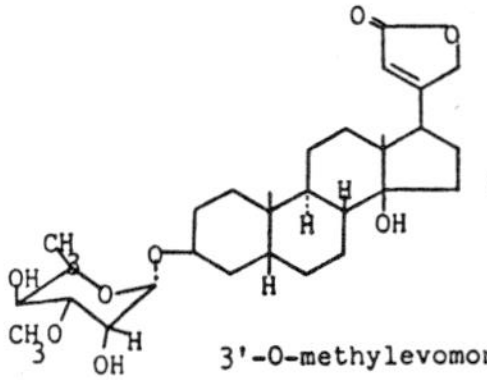 3'-O-methylevomonoside	inhibits KB cells at 2.7 x 10^{-3} μg/ml ED_{50} = 20 mg/kg	169
Allamanda cathartica 軟枝黃蟬花	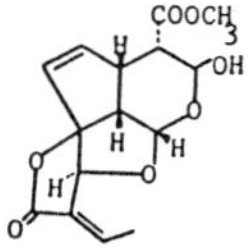 Allamandin	against P-388	142
Asclepiadaceae			
Asclepias curassavica 馬利筋	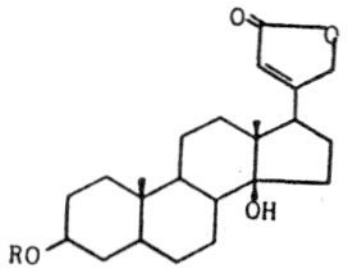 Uzarigenin R=H	A 50% aqueous ethanol extract inhibits KB in cell culture the active dosage is 1-3.5 μg/ml for KB, for P-388, 15-60 mg/kg	2, 79

Chinese Drugs and Related Plants Used to Treat Cancer

Plants	Active Principle	Anticancer Activity	Reference
Tylophora crebriflora 密花娃兒藤	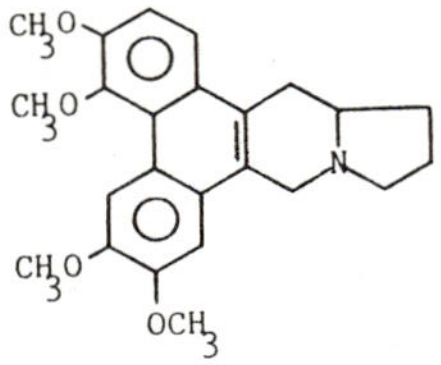 Tylophorine	CA-755, MS-lymphoma, WM-256, P-388, L-1210	131, 132
Wattakaka vobulili 烏骨藤		effective for Hodgkin's disease, gastric cancer, liver cancer	
Marsdenia tenacissima 烏骨藤	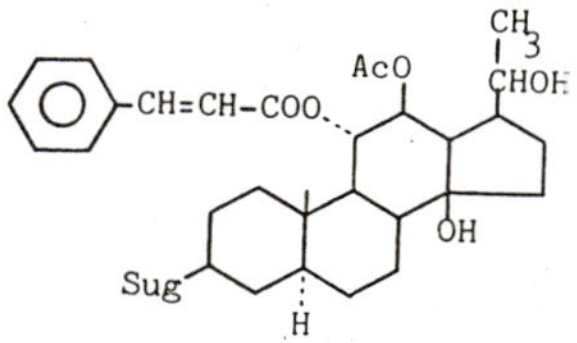		
M. cundurango 牛嬭菜		against S-180 and Ehrlich carcinoma	170
Cynanchum paniculatum Kitagawa (*Pycnostelma paniculatum* (Bunge) K. (Schum.) 徐長卿			
C. vincetokicum 藥用白前	Contains tylophorine		167

Chinese Drugs and Related Plants Used to Treat Cancer

Plants	Active Principle	Anticancer Activity	Reference
Berberidaceae			
Mahonia bealei Carr. (*M. fortunei* Moull.) 十大功勞			2
Podophyllum pleianthum 八角蓮	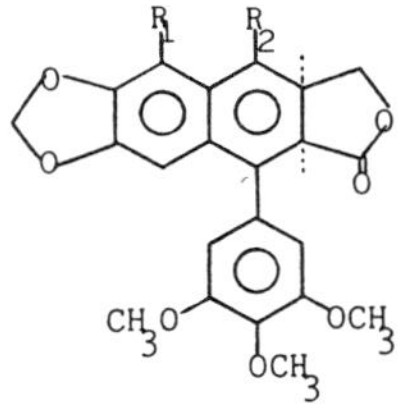 Podophyllotoxin	Ehrlich ascites, L-1210	171
P. peltatum 盾葉鬼臼	R_1=H R_2=OH		172
P. emodii 西艾鬼臼			173
P. sikkimensis	Podophyllotoxin derivatives		172
Betulaceae			
Alnus oregana Nutt 榿木	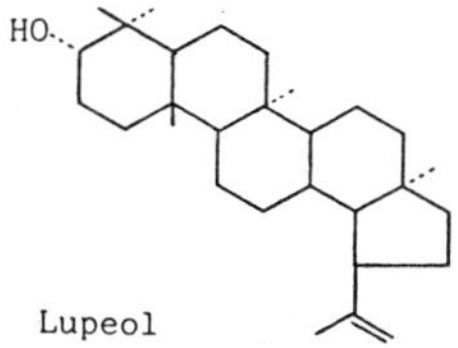 Lupeol	inhibits WM-256	174

Chinese Drugs and Related Plants Used to Treat Cancer

Plants	Active Principle	Anticancer Activity	Reference
Biognoniaceae *Acanthospermum glabratum* 刺苞菊	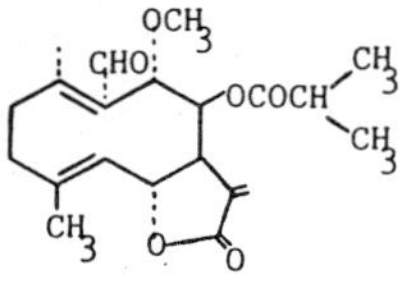 Acanthospermolide	ED_{50} = 0.54 μg/ml to KB cell; = 12 mg/kg to P-388	175
Tabebuia cassinoides	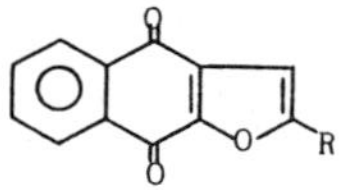 R=$COCH_3$ R=$CH(OH)CH_3$	the chloroform extract showed activity in P-388 assay (T/C=132 at 50 mg/kg); KB: ED_{50} = 1.2 μg/ml	176 91
Stereospermum suareolens		against WM-256, Ehrlich ascites, MS-lymphoma	177
S. tetragonum 羽葉楸	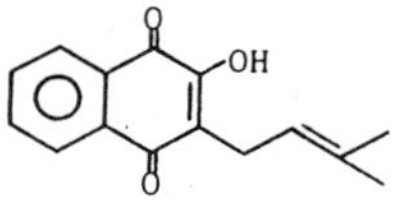 Lapachol		
Blasaminaceae *Impatients balsamina* 鳳仙花			

Chinese Drugs and Related Plants Used to Treat Cancer

Plants	Active Principle	Anticancer Activity	Reference
Boraginaceae *Arnebia nobillis* *A. thomsonii* 新疆紫草	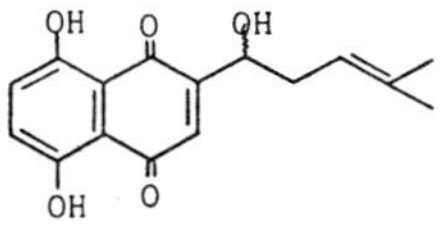 Alkannin (α-OH), Shikonin (β-OH)	against ascites cell of sarcoma-180 at a dose of 10 mg/kg	94
Burseraceae *Bursera microphylla* 小葉裂欖	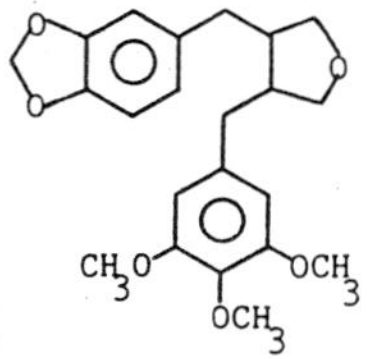 Burseran	KB $ED_{50} \leqslant 10$ mcg/ml	178
Campanulaceae *Lobelia chinensis* 半邊蓮			2

Chinese Drugs and Related Plants Used to Treat Cancer

Plants	Active Principle	Anticancer Activity	Reference
Celastraceae *Tripterygium wilfordii* 雷公藤	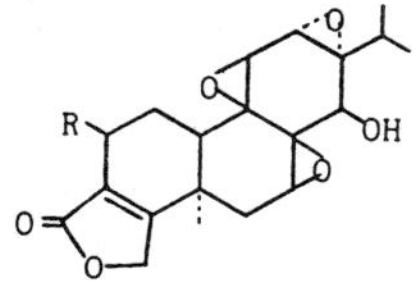 (I) R=H, (II) R=OH 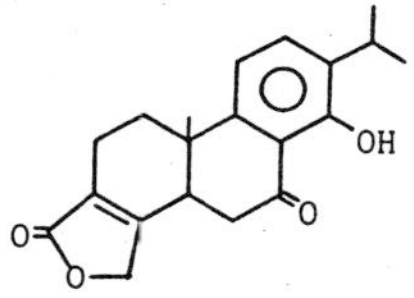 (III) 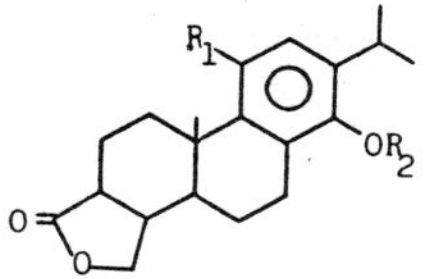 (IV) $R_1=R_2=H$ (V) $R_1=H$, $R_2=CH_3$ (VI) $R_1=OH$, $R_2=CH_3$ Triptolide (I), tripdiolide (II) triptonolide (III), triptophenol (IV), triptophenolide methylether (V), neotriptophenolide (VI)	triptolide at 0.1 mg/kg showed impressive life-prolonging effects (T/C ⩾ 230) in mice aflicted with L-1210 lymphoid leukemia	43, 179
Maytanus guangsiensis 廣西美登木 *M. hookeri* 美登木	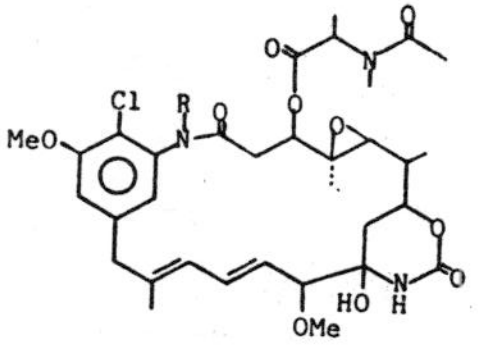 Maytansine R=CH_3 Normaytansine R=H	significantly inhibits P-388, S-180, Lewis lung cancer, L-1210, WM-256 at dosage level of μg/kg, $ED_{50} = 10^{-4} - 10^{-5}$ μg/ml against KB cell	152-159

Chinese Drugs and Related Plants Used to Treat Cancer

Plants	Active Principle	Anticancer Activity	Reference
Cephalotaxaceae *Cephalotaxus harringtonia* var. *clrupacea* 粗榧 *C. hainanensis*	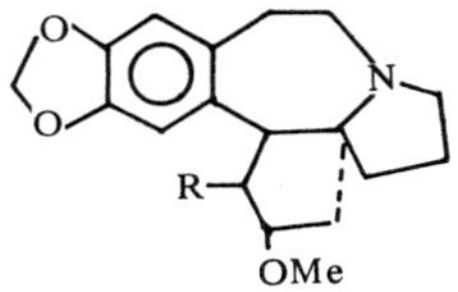	inhibits S-180, Walker-256 as well as P-388 the inhibition rate: S-180: 22-60% at 1-1.5 mg/kg; solid-type liver cancer: 32-44%; WM-256: 80.4%	122-125
C. fortunei 三尖杉 *C. sinensis* 中國粗榧 *C. omeii* 篦子尖杉 *C. wilsoniana* 台灣尖杉	(I) R = CH_2-C(OH)(CH_3)–$(CH_2)_2$-C(OH)(CO_2–)-$CH_2CO_2CH_3$ Harringtonine (I) Isoharringtonine Homoharringtonine	clinical application: lymphoma, Hodgkin's disease, choriocarcinoma, primary liver cancer and leukemia	
C. hainanensis 海南島尖杉	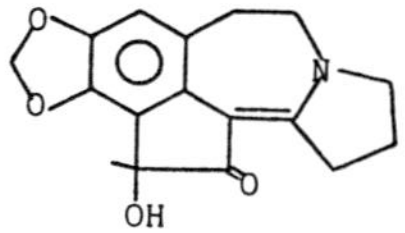 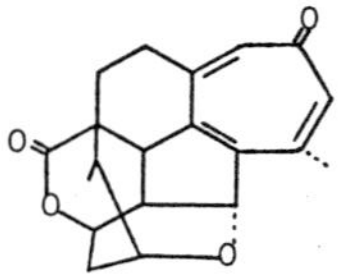 Hainanensis (I) Hainanolide (II)	effective against P-388	
Chloranthraceae *Sarcandra glaber* 九節茶	Flavone Glucosides	inhibits the growth of ascites sarcoma-180 cells *in vitro*	180

Chinese Drugs and Related Plants Used to Treat Cancer

Plants	Active Principle	Anticancer Activity	Reference
Compositae			
Artemisia vulgaris 眞蘄艾			2
Eclipta alba 旱蓮草			2
Elephantopus elatus	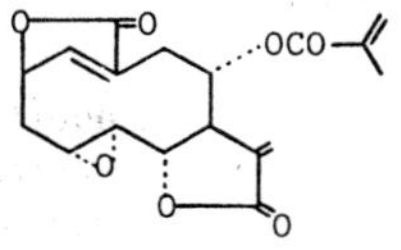 Elephantopin	KB ED_{50} = 0.3 μg/ml P-388 T/C = 171% at 40 mg/kg, L-1210	11, 181
E. scaber 丁茄柕	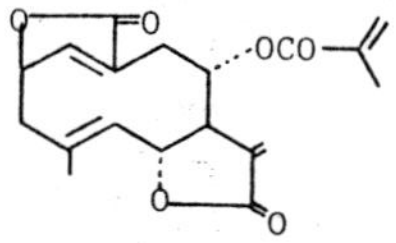 Deoxoelephantopin		
E. mollis 地膽草	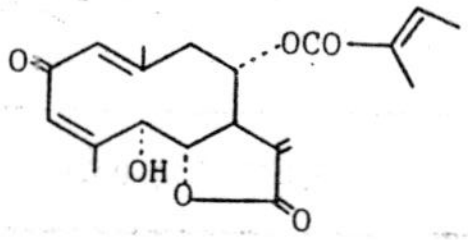 Molephantinin	WM-256, T/C = 397% at 2.5 mg/kg/day in rats; also active against P-388, and Ehrlich ascites growth	12

Chinese Drugs and Related Plants Used to Treat Cancer

Plants	Active Principle	Anticancer Activity	Reference
Eupatorium rotundifolium 圓葉澤蘭	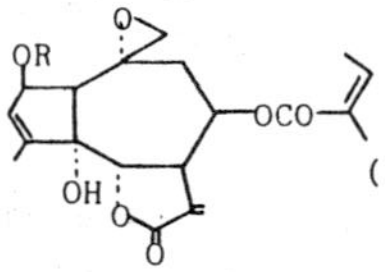 (I) R=H (II) R=Ac Euparotin (I) Euparotin acetate (II)	KB ED_{50} = 0.21 μg/ml	182, 183
Centaurea hyssopifolia 矢車菊屬	Cynaropicrin (I) Deacylcynaropicrin (II)	against HeLa cell	188
C. linifolia	Chlorohyssopifolin-A (III), -B (IV), C (V), -D (VI)		
Chloranthus japonicus 金粟蘭	Chloranthalactone-A (VII), -B (VIII)	against rat lymphoma, L-5178y	5
Helenium microcephatum 堆心菊	Helenalin, microhelenin E (IX)	antileukemic activity	197

Chinese Drugs and Related Plants Used to Treat Cancer

Plants	Active Principle	Anticancer Activity	Reference
Pertya robusta 帚菊	Glucozaluzanin (X) (VII) (VIII) (I) $R_1R_2=CH_2$, $R_3=\overset{O}{\overset{\Vert}{C}}-C(=CH_2)CH_2OH$ (II) $R_1R_2=CH_2$, $R_3=H$ (III) $R_1=CH_2Cl$, $R_2=OH$ $R_3=\overset{O}{\overset{\Vert}{C}}-C(OH)(CH_3)CH_2Cl$ (IV) $R_1=CH_2Cl$, $R_2=OH$, $R_3=H$ (V) $R_1R_2=-O-CH_2-$ $R_3=\overset{O}{\overset{\Vert}{C}}C(OH)(CH_3)CH_2Cl$ (VI) $R_1=R_2=H$, $R_3=\overset{O}{\overset{\Vert}{C}}-C(CH_3)(OC_2H_5)-CH_2OH$ (IX) (X)	cytotoxicity	189

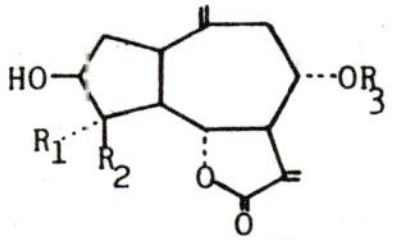

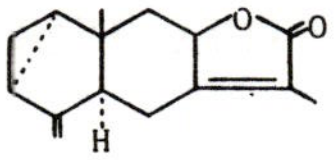

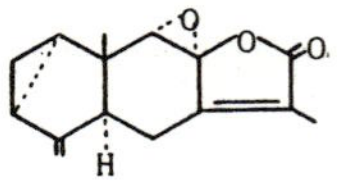

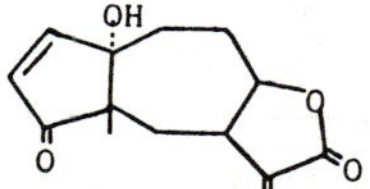

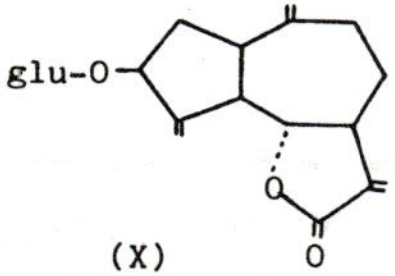

Chinese Drugs and Related Plants Used to Treat Cancer

Plants	Active Principle	Anticancer Activity	Reference
Eupatorium formosanum Hay. 台灣澤蘭	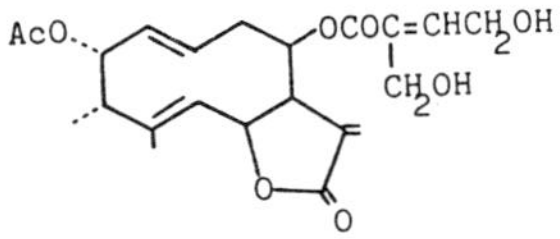 AcO, OCOC=CHCH$_2$OH, CH$_2$OH, O Eupaformosanin	inhibits WM-256, P-388, Ehrlich ascites, and Lewis lung tumor	3
Gaillardia pulchella 天人菊	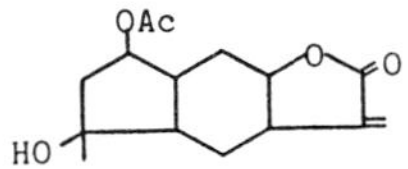 OAc, HO, O Gaillardin	against KB ED_{50} = 2.30 μg/ml *in vitro*	184
Gutierrezia sarothrae 古堆菊	Saccharide-protein	inhibits sarcoma-180	185
Vernonia hymenolepsis 斑鳩菊 *V. andersonii* 過山龍	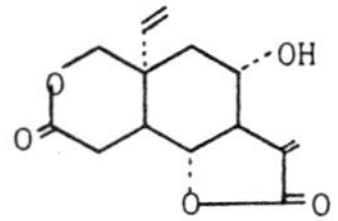 OH, O Vernolepin Methacrylate Vernolepin (I) Vernonine	KB ED_{50} = 0.42 μg/ml KB ED_{50} = 2.0 μg/ml	186

Chinese Drugs and Related Plants Used to Treat Cancer

Plants	Active Principle	Anticancer Activity	Reference
Ligularia tussilaginea 活血蓮			2
Senecio kirilowii 狗血草	Pyrrolizidine alkaloids		2
Senecio fendeleri	Wedeliatoxin	against leukemia T/C = 120% at 5 mg/kg	88
Wedelia asperrima	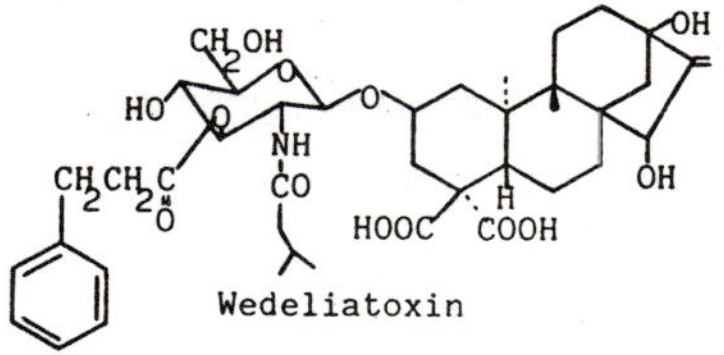	against the carcinogenic action of aflatoxin B, LD_{50} = 1 mg/kg	187
Cupressaceae			
Juniperus phoenicea 腓尼基檜	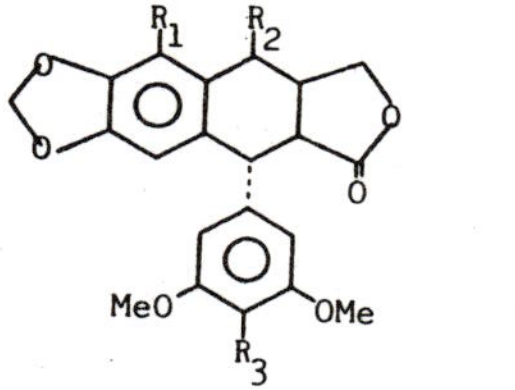 (I) $R_1=OCH_3$, $R_2=H$, $R_3=OCH_3$ (II) $R_1=R_2=H$, $R_3=OCH_3$ β-peltatin-A-methyl ether (I) Desoxypodophyllotoxin (II)	against P-388	190

Chinese Drugs and Related Plants Used to Treat Cancer

Plants	Active Principle	Anticancer Activity	Reference
Cucurbitaceae			
Melothria heterophylla 杜爪根	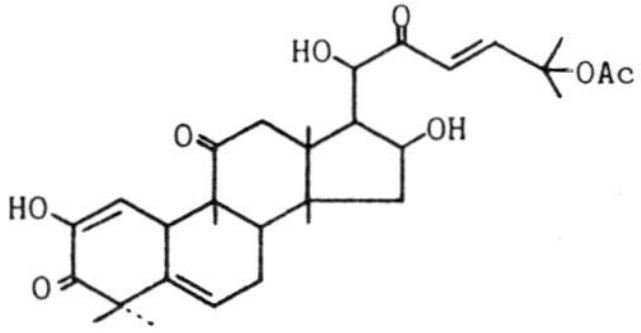 Cucurbitacines		2, 167
Dioscoreaceae			
Dioscorea bulbifera 黄藥子		inhibits Ehrlich ascites cell and sarcoma-180	2
Euphorbiaceae			
Croton crassifolius			
C. macrostachys 長穗巴豆	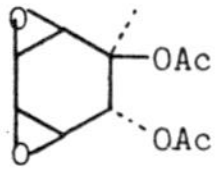 Crotepoxide		191
Euphorbia helioscopia 澤漆			
Jatropha cinecis L. 麻風樹	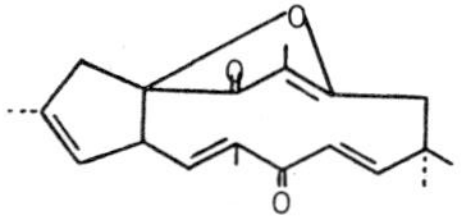		192

Chinese Drugs and Related Plants Used to Treat Cancer

Plants	Active Principle	Anticancer Activity	Reference
J. gossypifolia 棉葉麻風樹 *J. multifida* 珊瑚花 *J. podagrica* 佛杜樹		inhibits sarcoma-180, WM-256, P-388, Lewis cancer, and KB	192
Micrandra elata	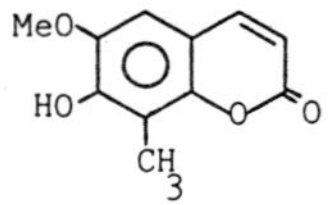 Isofrexidin	P-388, ED_{50} = 1.7 μg/ml	193
Ricinum communis 蓖麻	Ricin (protein)	inhibits Ehrlich ascites	194
Geraniaceae			
Pelargonium geraveolens 香葉天竺葵	Volatile oil	*in vitro,* inhibits the growth of HeLa cell and Ec-cancer; *in vivo,* shows an inhibitory action against transplanted S-37, S-180, Ehrlich ascites cells, and WM-256, with total effective rate of 70.4% for the treatment of cervical cancer.	6

Chinese Drugs and Related Plants Used to Treat Cancer

Plants	Active Principle	Anticancer Activity	Reference
Gramineae *Coix lachryma* 薏苡	$CH_3-CH-O-CO-C(CH_2)_9-CH=CH-(CH_2)_5-CH_3$ $CH_3-CH-O-CO-C(CH_2)_7-CH=CH-(CH_2)_5-CH_3$ Coixenolide	against U-14, Ehrlich ascites cells	195
Iridaceae *Iris pallasii* var. *chinensis* 馬蘭子	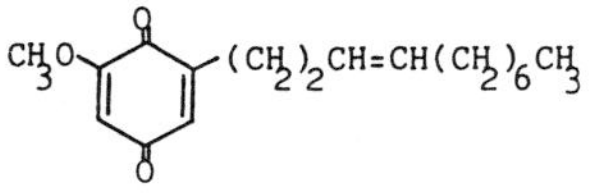 Irisquinone	marked efficacy to the cervical cancer U-14 in mice, and also showed inhibitory action against liver cancer, lymphoma, and Ehrlich carcinoma	11
Hydrocharitaceae *Trapa bicornus* Okbeck (*T. japonica* Flerov)			2
Juglandaceae *Juglans regia* 黑胡桃 *J. nigra*	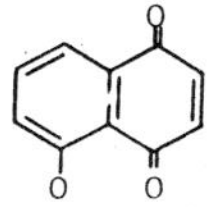 Juglone	Ehrlich ascites and autonomic adenoma of rats	196

Chinese Drugs and Related Plants Used to Treat Cancer

Plants	Active Principle	Anticancer Activity	Reference
Labiatae			
Rabdonia rubescens (*Isodon rubescens*) 冬凌草	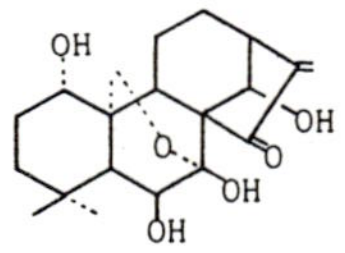 Oridonin (I) 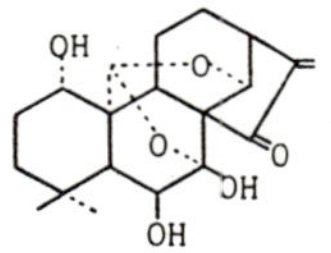 Ponicidin (II)	for the treatment of late stages of cancer of the esophagus Oridonin inhibits DNA synthesis of Ehrlich carcinoma	11,63-65
Isodon amethystoides 王棗子	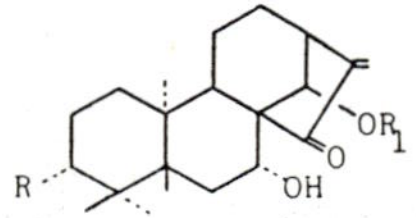 Amethytodin A, B, C Oridonin (A) R=OH, R_1=H (B) R==O, R_1=H (C) R==O, R_1=Ac	inhibits S-180, Ehrlich ascites at dose of 20 mg/kg	45
I. longitubus 長管香茶菜	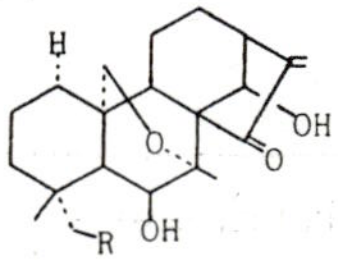 (A) R=11 (B) R=OAc Longikaurin A and B	*in vitro* inhibits breast cancer FM 3A/B cell of mice	72

Chinese Drugs and Related Plants Used to Treat Cancer

Plants	Active Principle	Anticancer Activity	Reference
Roylea calycina	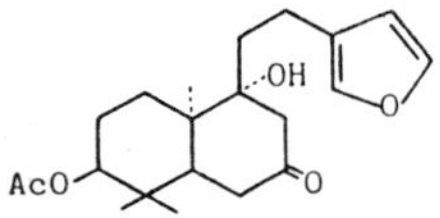 Precalyone	against P-388, T/C = 143 at 50 mg/kg	198
Salvia przewalskii var. *mandarinorum* 紫丹參	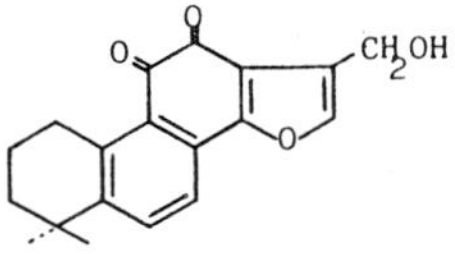 Przewaquinone A	the inhibition rate is 35.8-67.8% to Lewis lung cancer, melanoma, and S-180 at 120-150 mg/kg in mice	99
Scutellaria barbata 半枝蓮			2
Lardizabalaceae			
Akebia trifoliata 八月札			2
Sargentodoxa cuneata 紅藤			2
Lauraceae			
Nectandra rigida	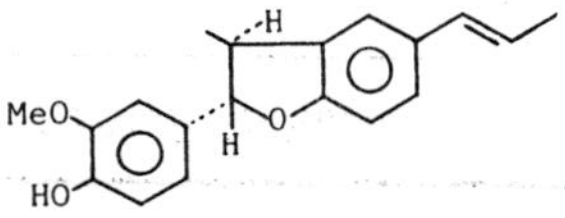 Licarin	inhibits KB cells	199

Chinese Drugs and Related Plants Used to Treat Cancer

Plants	Active Principle	Anticancer Activity	Reference
Leguminosae *Crotalaria retusa* *C. assamica* 大葉猪屎豆 *C. sessiliflora* 農吉利 *C. spectabilis* 美麗猪屎豆	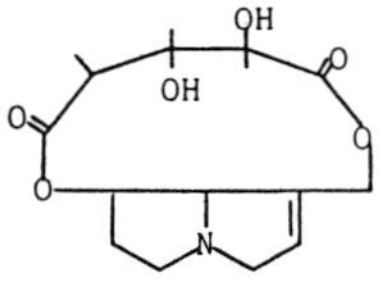 Monocrotaline (1) Spectabiline Senecionine	WM-256, S-180, CA-755 monocrotaline has been used for treating skin cancer	143-151
Heliotropium lasiocarpum 天芥菜 (Boraginaceae)	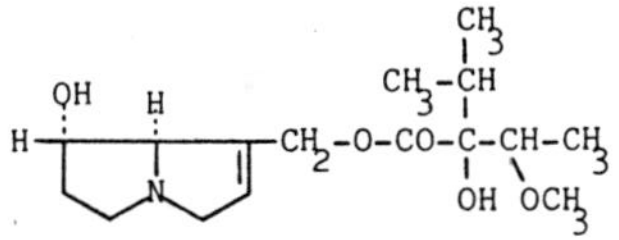 Heliotrine (1) Lasiocarpine	WM-256, L-1210, P-388, P-1535, melanoma-B-16	143
H. indicum (Boraginaceae) 大尾摇	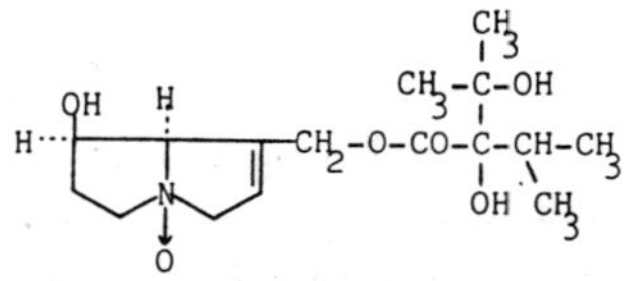 Indicine-N-oxide	similar to heliotrine	144

Chinese Drugs and Related Plants Used to Treat Cancer

Plants	Active Principle	Anticancer Activity	Reference
Pterocarpus indicus 青龍木 *Sophora subprostrata* 廣豆根	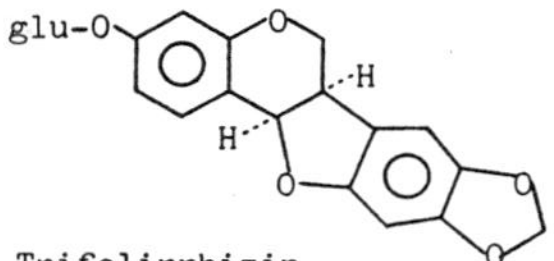 glu-O (structure) Trifolirrhizin	Ehrlich ascites	236
S. flavescens 苦參	Matrine, Oxymatrine 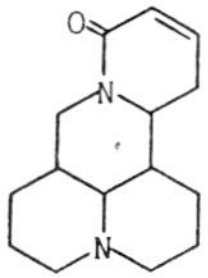 Matrine and Oxymatrine (N→O)	against Ehrlich ascites, S-180 uses: gastric cancer, liver cancer, cervix cancer	200
S. japonica 山豆根 *Euchresta japonica* 山豆根			11, 166
Sophora alopecuroides 苦豆子	Sophocarpine	inhibits S-180	236

Chinese Drugs and Related Plants Used to Treat Cancer

Plants	Active Principle	Anticancer Activity	Reference
Sophora flavescens 苦參	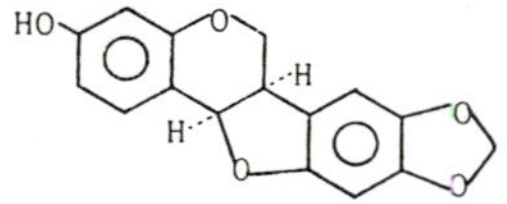 l-maackianin	inhibits S-180	236
S. japonica 槐樹	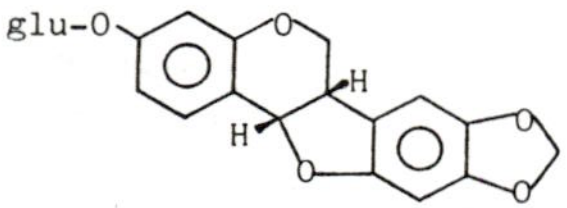 Sophojaponicin	inhibits S-180	236
Dolichos fulculus 鐮果扁豆		inhibits several kind of animal tumor systems	200
Sesbania drummodii 田菁	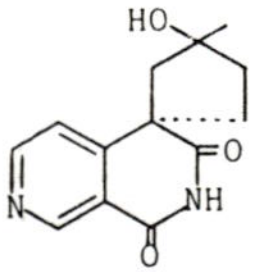 Sesbanine 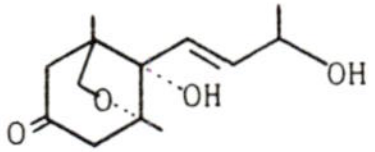 Drummondol	cytotoxicity	201
Desmodium styraeifolium 金錢草			2
Lespedeza cuneata 火魚草			2
Wisteria floribunda 紫藤瘤			2

Chinese Drugs and Related Plants Used to Treat Cancer

Plants	Active Principle	Anticancer Activity	Reference
Liliaceae			
Colchicum autumnale 秋水仙 *Iphigenia indica* A Gray. 山慈菇	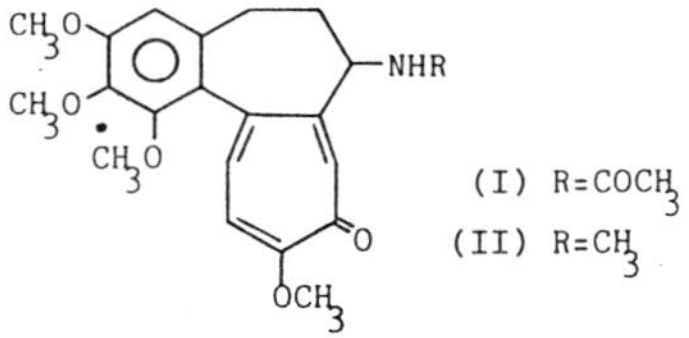 (I) R=$COCH_3$ (II) R=CH_3 Colchicine (I), Demecolcine (II)	against L-1210, CA-755, S-180, S-37, WM-256 use: skin cancer, chronic leukemia	202, 203
Paris polyphylla 七葉一枝花	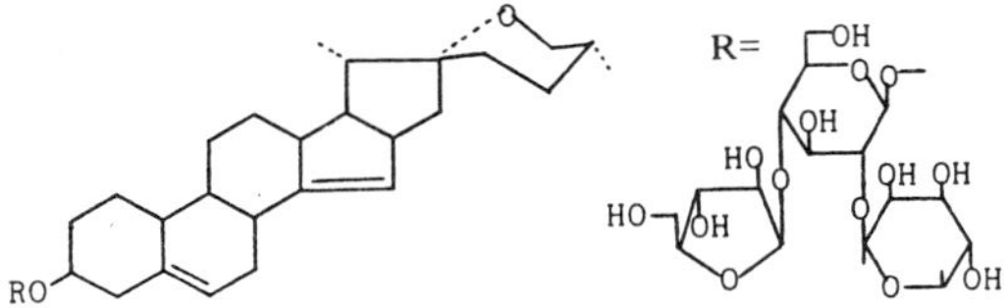 R=	against P-388, L-1210, KB cell, ED_{50} = 0.94, 0.14, 0.16 μg/ml, respectively	204
Smilax china 金剛藤			2
Loranthaceae			
Viscum album			
V. coloratum 槲寄生	Viscotoxin A	Sarcoma-180	205

Chinese Drugs and Related Plants Used to Treat Cancer

Plants	Active Principle	Anticancer Activity	Reference
Magnoliaceae *Michelia compressa* 烏心石	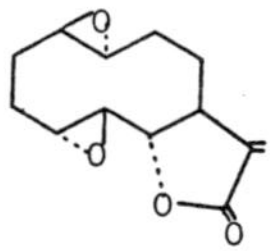 Michelenolide (I) 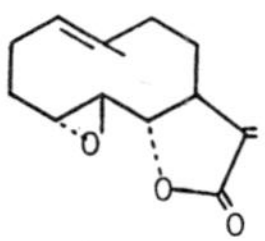 Parthenolide (II)	*in vitro* inhibits WM-256 and KB	3
Malvaceae *Hibiscus mutabilis* 木芙蓉			2
Melastomataceae *Melastoma candidum* 野牡丹			2
Meloidae *Mylabris phalerate* Pall 大斑蝥 *M. cichorri* 小斑蝥	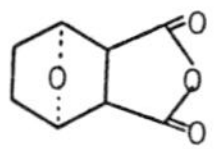 Cantharidin	prolongs the survival of patients with liver cancer	11

Chinese Drugs and Related Plants Used to Treat Cancer

Plants	Active Principle	Anticancer Activity	Reference
Menispermaceae			
Stephania tetrandra 漢防己 *S. hernandiflora* 千金藤 *Cyclea* genera 輪環藤屬 *Menispermum* genera 蝙蝠葛屬	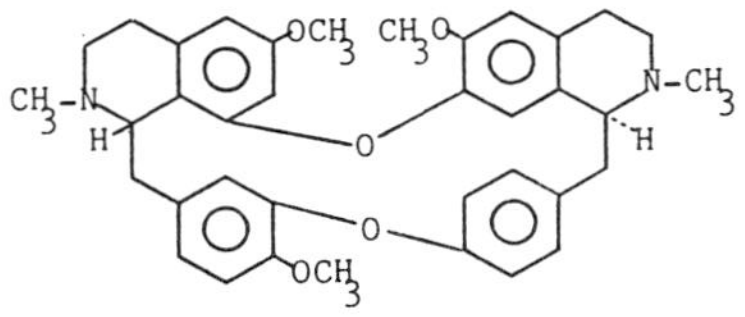 tetradrine	against WM-256 and KB cells	80, 206
Moraceae			
Ficus pumila 薜荔果	β-amyrine ester		
F. septica	Tylocrebrine alkaloids	CA-755, MS-lymphoma, WM-256, P-388, L-1210	2
Humulus japonicus Sieb. et Zucc. *(H. scandens* Lour. Merr.*)* 葎草	Vitexine		2

Chinese Drugs and Related Plants Used to Treat Cancer

Plants	Active Principle	Anticancer Activity	Reference
Maclura aurantic	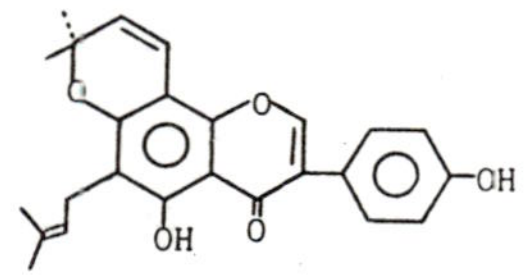 Osayin	against Ehrlich ascites, S-37, S-180, WM-256	
Myrsinaceae			
Ardisia crenata 大羅傘			2
A. japonica 紫金牛			2
Nyctaginaceae			
Mirabilis multiflora	Saccharide-proteins	S-180, WM-256, Lewis lung cancer, lymphomas	207, 208
Nyssaceae			
Camptotheca acuminata Decaisue 喜樹	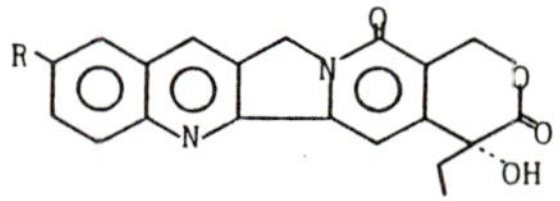 Camptothecine R=H Hydroxycamptothecine R=OH	inhibits CA-755, L-1210, WM-256 clinical uses: gastrointestinal carcinomas and leukemia	11, 209, 210

Chinese Drugs and Related Plants Used to Treat Cancer

Plants	Active Principle	Anticancer Activity	Reference
Palmaceae			
Livistona chinensis 葵樹子			2
Polygonaceae			
Polygonum cuspidatum 虎杖	Piceid, polidalin		2
P. cymosum 開金鎖			
P. orientale 水紅花子	Emodin 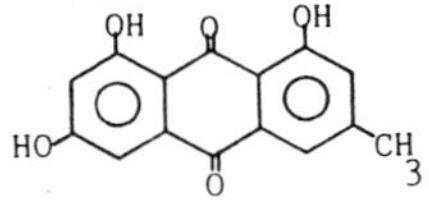	against lymphocytic leukemia in mice	211
Rumex madaio 土大黃	Deuticulatol		2
Polypodiaceae			
Microsorium hancockii 綠鷄尾			2
Pteris multifida 鳳尾草			2
Polyporaceae			
Polyporus umbellatus 猪苓	Polysaccharide	against sarcoma-180; clinical study has shown an immuno-stimulating action	212

Chinese Drugs and Related Plants Used to Treat Cancer

Plants	Active Principle	Anticancer Activity	Reference
Ganoderma lucidum 靈芝	Polysaccharide	strongly inhibited the growth of sarcoma-180, with inhibition rate of 95.6-98.6% at a dosage of 20 mg/kg for 10 days in mice, I.P.	213
Poria cocos 茯苓	Polysaccharides	increases the curative effect of antitumor agents, and shows immuno-stimulating action	214
Letinus edodes 香菇	Polysaccharides	markedly inhibits growth of sarcoma-180 in mice	215, 216
Ranunculaceae			
Adonis amurensis 福壽草	strophanthidin and its glucoside	ED_{50} = 0.25 μg/ml in cell culture against carcinoma of nasopharynx	80
Clematis florida 鐵線草			2

Chinese Drugs and Related Plants Used to Treat Cancer

Plants	Active Principle	Anticancer Activity	Reference
Thalictrum dasycarpum 紫唐松草 *T. minus* 小唐松草 *T. minus* var. *elatrum* 匈牙利唐松草 *T. fendleri* 芬德勒氏唐松草 *T. revolatum*	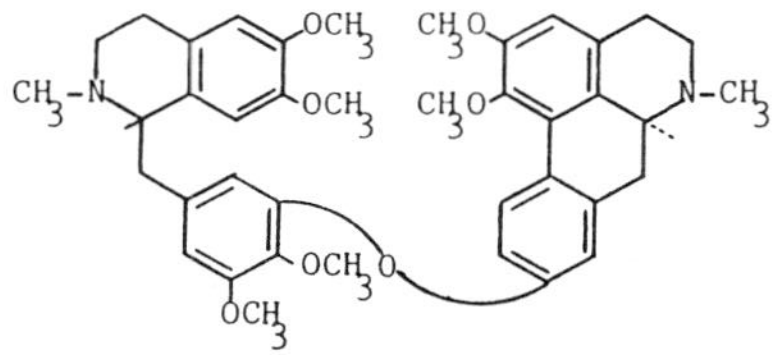 Thalicarpine	inhibits WM-256, Lewis lung cancer and KB cells against WM-256, therapeutic index > 4	217
Rosaceae			
Duchesnea indica 蛇莓			2
Rubiaceae			
Adina pilulifera (*A. rubella* Hance) 水楊梅根			2
Galium aparine 猪殃殃			2
Hedyotis chrysotricha 石打穿			2

Chinese Drugs and Related Plants Used to Treat Cancer

Plants	Active Principle	Anticancer Activity	Reference
Oldenlandia diffusa 白花蛇舌草	Iriroids and β-sitosterols	stimulates proliferation of the reticuloendothelial system and intensifies the phagocytosis of phagocyte	218, 219
Rondeletia panamensis	HO, O, H, H Panamensin HO, O, O, H, H, OH Oxidopanamensin	inhibits KB cell at 2.6 and 1.9 μg/ml, respectively	5
Cephaelis ipecacuanha 吐根	CH_3O, CH_3O, NH, OCH_3, OCH_3, N Emetin	against L-1210, melanoma B-16, P-388 clinical uses: chronic granulocytic leukemia, lympho-reticulocytoma, rectal cancer, cystic carcinoma, and lingua carcinoma	221, 222

Chinese Drugs and Related Plants Used to Treat Cancer

Plants	Active Principle	Anticancer Activity	Reference
Morinda parvifolia Bart. 百眼藤	Morindaparin A	*in vivo*, T/C = 152% at 50 mg/kg/day I.P. in P-388; with ED_{50} = 1.85 μg/ml against the *in vitro* growth of P-388	135
Rutaceae			
Acronychia baueri Schoff 鮑爾氏山柚柑 *A. oligophlebia* 貢甲 *A. peduncudata* 降眞香	Acronycine	acronycine has a broad spectrum of antitumor activity and showed significant inhibitory action on 12 kinds among 17 kinds of animal tumor systems tested, including C-1498, X-5563, and Shionogi carcinoma-115	129, 130
Zanthoxylum nitidum 兩面針	Nitidine chloride	exhibited antileukemic activity in both leukemic L-1210 and P-388 systems	137-139

Chinese Drugs and Related Plants Used to Treat Cancer

Plants	Active Principle	Anticancer Activity	Reference
Selaginellaceae *Selaginella doederleinii* 石上柏	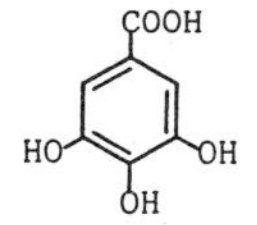 Shikimic acid	possesses cytotoxic activity	223
			2
S. moellendorfii 岩柏			
Simaroubaceae *Ailanthus grandis* 臭椿	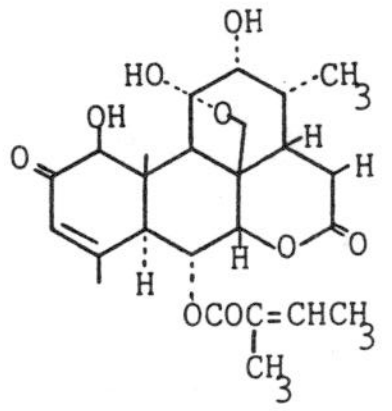 6-Tigloyloxychaparrinone	P-388; ED_{50} = 0.01 μg/ml	11
Brucea javanica 鴉膽子	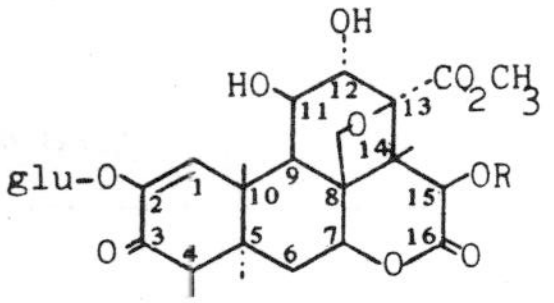 Bruceoside-A R=-COCHC< (I) Brusatol (II) 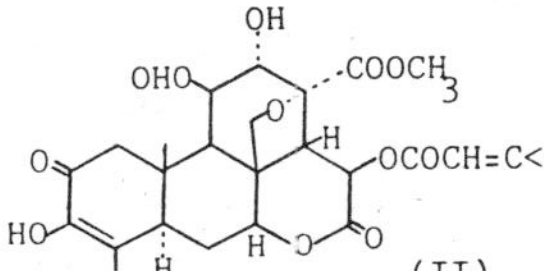	possesses significant antileukemic activity in P-388 lymphocytic leukemia with T/C > 120%	20-23

Chinese Drugs and Related Plants Used to Treat Cancer

Plants	Active Principle	Anticancer Activity	Reference
Solanaceae			
Physalis minima 燈籠草 *P. fraucheti* 酸漿	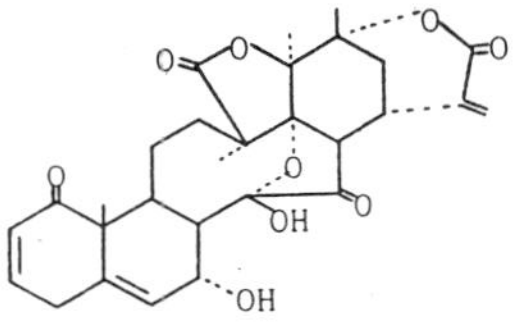Physalin-A		167, 224
P. alkekengi var. *fraucheti*			
Solanum lyratum 白英			2
S. dulcamara L. 千年不爛心，蜀羊泉	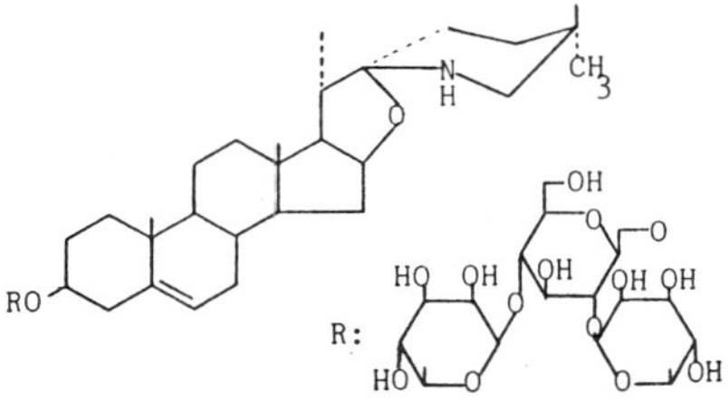β-solamarine	β-solamarine markedly inhibits the growth of S-180 and WM-256. Crude drugs are folklore remedy for tumors and warts in many countries.	225
S. nigrum 龍葵			2
S. nidicum 紫花茄			71
S. verbasifolium 洗碗葉			

Chinese Drugs and Related Plants Used to Treat Cancer

Plants	Active Principle	Anticancer Activity	Reference
S. tripartitum	$(CH_3)_2N-(CH_2)_4$ / $(CH_3)_2N-(CH_2)_4$ >N-C(=O)-CH=CH(CH$_2$)$_{12}$CH$_3$ Solapalmitenine	WM-256	226
Taxaceae *Taxus chinensis* 紅豆杉 *T. baceata* 漿果紫杉 *T. brevifolia* 短葉紫杉 *T. cuspidata* 東北紫杉 *T. speciosa* 南方紅豆杉 *T. yunnanensis* 雲南紅豆杉	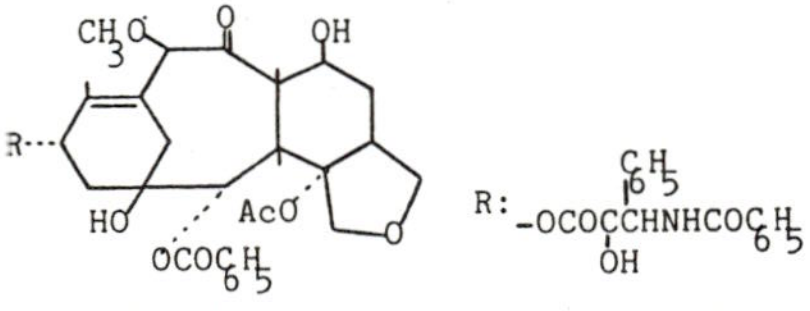 Taxol R: $-OCOCH(C_6H_5)CH(OH)NHCOC_6H_5$	against P-388, P-1534, WM-256, S-180, L-1210, Lewis lung cancer, KB cells	227
Taxodiaceae *Taxodium distichum* 落羽杉	Taxodione Taxodone (R= α-OH) 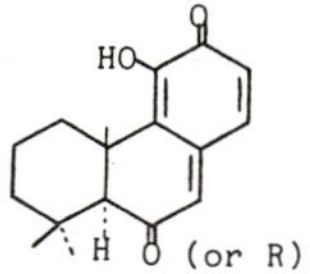	WM-256	228

Chinese Drugs and Related Plants Used to Treat Cancer

Plants	Active Principle	Anticancer Activity	Reference
Podocarpus milanjianus 羅漢松	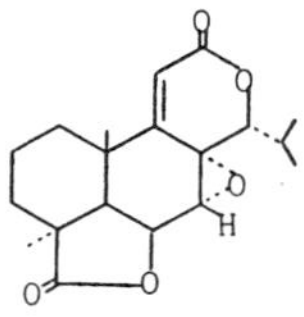 Nagilactone G, 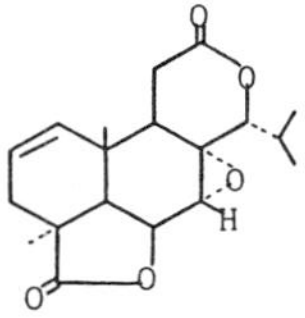 Milangilactone A, 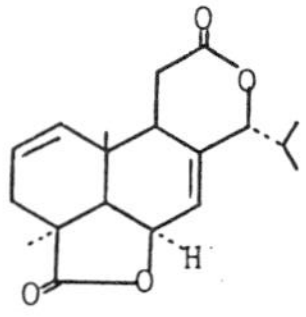 Milangilactone B	against KB cell	229, 230
Thymelaeaceae *Daphne genkwa* 芫花 *D. odorata* 瑞香	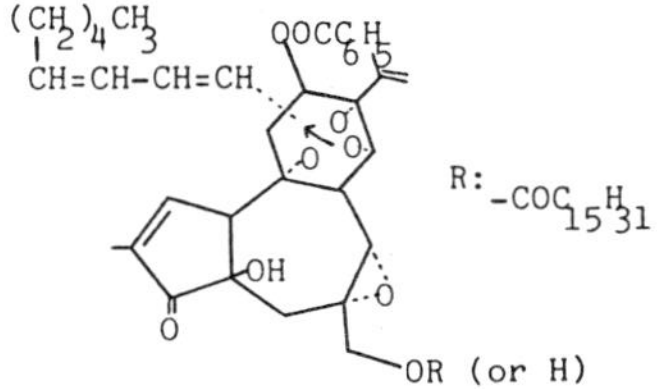 Gnidilatidin and its ester (R: $-COC_{15}H_{31}$; OR (or H))	antileukemic action	77
Wikstroemia indica 了哥王	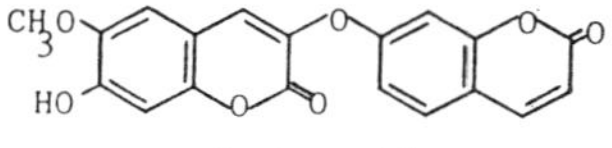 Daphnoretin 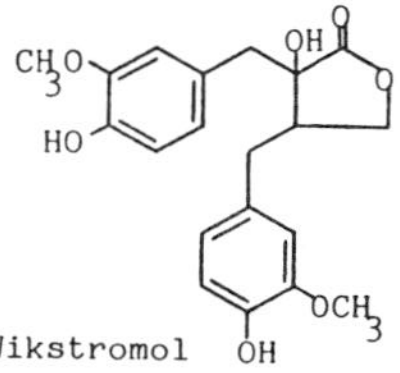 Wikstromol	significantly inhibits Ehrlich ascites carcinoma growth at dose of 3-12 mg/kg	231, 232, 233
		P-388: T/C = 146% at 10 mg/kg	234

Chinese Drugs and Related Plants Used to Treat Cancer

Plants	Active Principle	Anticancer Activity	Reference
Usneaceae			
Usnea diffracta Vain (*U. longissima* Ach.) 松蘿	Usnic acid		2
Valerianaceae			
Patrinia heterophylla 墓回頭			2
P. villosa 敗醬			
Valeriana walliahii	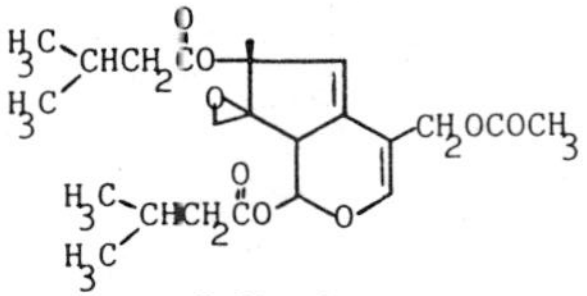 Valtrate	*in vitro* inhibits liver cancer of mice; *in vivo* effective against KREBS II tumor	235
Verbenaceae			
Verbena officinalis 馬鞭草			2
Violaceae			
Viola collina 黄瓜香			2

Chinese Drugs and Related Plants Used to Treat Cancer

Plants	Active Principle	Anticancer Activity	Reference
Vitaceae *Ampelopsis brevipedunculata* 野葡萄			2
Zingiberaceae *Curcuma aromatica* 莪朮	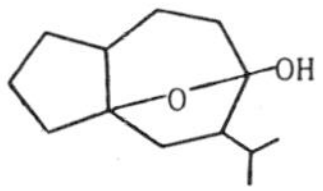 Curcumol and 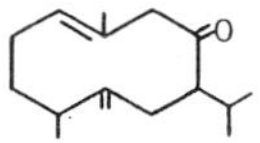 curdione	shows an inhibitory effect on sarcoma-180 in mice. This drug has been used for the treatment of the early stage of cervical cancer.	11

10. Summary

Over 120 species of plants belonging to some 60 different families have been used either in Chinese traditional or folk medicine to treat cancer. Selected examples of these plants with established chemistry and known pharmacology are presented. The structural requirements for bioactive sesquiterpenes, diterpenes, triterpenes, steroids, and alkaloids are examined. Primary biochemical targets of some of these anticancer activities of the anticancer Chinese plants and related species are compiled. Special emphasis is placed on the potential uses as well as possible side effects and toxicities based on the current knowledge of structure-activity relationships.

11. References

1. M. Suffness and J. Douros, *J. Nat. Products* 45(1): 1-14 (1982).
2. H. Y. Hsu, *Treating Cancer with Chinese Herbs,* Oriental Healing Arts Institute, Los Angeles, pp. 205-240, 1982.
3. H. Y. Hsu, Y. P. Chen, and N. M. Hong, *Chemistry of Chinese Herb Drugs,* Vol. 2, Brion Research Institute of Taiwan, Taipei, 1979.
4. J. H. Chen, F. P. Ea, S. C. Loa, P. J. Shai, M. L. Ding, and Z. N. Lu, *Zhong C'aoyao* 11(1): 1-14 (1980).
5. D. Y. Chu, *Zhong C'aoyao* 13(8): 41-48 (1982).
6. Y. H. Yau, *Yaoxue Tongbao* 16(7): 37 (1981).
7. B. A. Zhau and M. S. Wang, *Guwei Yaoxue, Zhiwu Yao Fengchie* 2(5): 1-5 (1981).
8. Y. Z. Wang and S. L. Zhong, *Yaoxue Xuebao* 18(1): 25-32 (1983).
9. R. W. Doskotch, C. D. Hufford, and F. S. El-Feraly, *J. Org. Chem.* 37: 2740-2744 (1972).
10. C. H. Smith, J. Larner, A. H. Thomas, and S. M. Kupchan, *Biochem. Biophys. Acta* 276: 94 (1972).
11. J. L. Beal and E. Reinhard, *Natural Products as Medicinal Agents,* Hippokrates, 1981.
12. I. H. Hall, Y. F. Liou, and K. H. Lee, *J. Pharm. Sci.* 71: 587-689 (1982).
13. S. M. Kupchan, M. A. Eakin, and T. J. Giacobbe, *Science* 168: 376-377 (1970); 168: 378-379 (1970).
14. K. H. Lee and H. Furukawa, *J. Med. Chem.* 15(6): 609-611 (1972).

15. I. H. Hall, K. H. Lee, E. C. Mar. and C. O. Starnes, *J. Med. Chem.* 20(3): 333-337 (1977).
16. K. H. Lee, *J. Pharm. Sci.* 62(6): 1028-1029 (1973).
17. S. M. Kupchan, R. W. Britton, J. A. Lacadie, M. F. Ziefler, and C. W. Sigel, *J. Org. Chem.* 40: 648-658 (1975).
18. S. M. Kupchan and J. A. Lacadie, *J. Org. Chem.* 38: 178 (1973).
19. J. D. Phillipson and F. A. Darwish, *Planta Medica* 35: 308-315 (1979).
20. K. H. Lee, Y. Imakura, Y. Sumida, R. Y. Wu, and I. H. Hall, *J. Org. Chem.* 44(13): 2180-2185 (1979).
21. J. D. Phillipson and F. A. Darwish, *Planta Medica* 41(3): 209-220 (1981).
22. J. S. Zhang,. L. Z. Lin, Z. L. Chen, and R. S. Xu, *Planta Medica* 39: 265 (1980).
23. L. Z. Lin, J. S. Zhang, Z. L. Chen, and R. S. Xu, *Huaxue Xuebao* 40(1): 73-78 (1982).
24. K. H. Lee, M. Okano, I. H. Hall, D. A. Brent, and B. Solmann, *J. Pharm. Sci.* 71(3): 338-345; 345-348 (1982).
25. O. D. Dailey, Jr. and P. L. Fuchs, *J. Org. Chem.*, 45: 216-236 (1980).
26. S. M. Kupchan and D. R. Streelman, *J. Org.* Chem., 41: 3481-3482 (1976).
27. M. Ohano and K. H. Lee, *J. Org. Chem.* 46: 1138-1141 (1981).
28. M. E. Wall and M. C. Wani, *J. Med. Chem.* 21(12): 1186-1187 (1978).
29. R. W. Doskotch, C. D. Hufford, and F. S. El-Feraly, *J. Org. Chem.* 37: 2740-2744 (1972).
30. E. Fujita, J. Magao, Y. Kanedo, S. Nakazama, and H. Kuroda, *Chem. Pharm. Bull.* 24: 2118-2127 (1976).
31. S. M. Kupchan and R. M. Schubert, *Science* 185: 791 (1974).
32. E. J. Lien, K. K. Hsu, and Y. C. Lin,. *J. Taiwan Pharm. Assoc.* 28: 22-26 (1976).
33. J. D. Phillipson and F. A. Laca Darwish, *Planta Medica* 35: 308-315 (1979).
34. S. M. Kupchan and J. A. Lacadie, *J. Org. Chem.* 40(5):

654-655 (1975).
35. J. Polousky, J. Varenne, T. Prange, and C. Pascard, *Tetrahedron Letters* 21: 1835-1836 (1980).
36. L. L. Liao, S. M. Kupchan, and S. B. Horwitz, *Molecular Pharmaco.* 12: 167-176 (1976).
37. M. Fresno, A. Gonzales, D. Vasquez, and A. Jimenez, *Biochem. et Biophys. Acta,* 518: 102-112 (1978).
38. Y. F. Liou, I. H. Hall, M. Okano, K. H. Lee, and S. G. Chaney, *J. Pharm. Sci.* 71(4): 430-435 (1982).
39. I. H. Hall, Y. F. Liou, K. H. Lee, M. Okano, and S. G. Chaney, *J. Pharm. Sci.* 71(2): 257-262 (1982).
40. A. Y. Bedikian, M. Valdivieso, G. P. Bodey, W. K. Marphy, and E. J. Freireich, *Cancer Treat. Rep.* 63: 1843-1847 (1979).
41. M. B. Garnick, R. H. Blum, G. P. Canellos, R. J. Mayer, L. Parker, A. T. Sharin, F. P. Li, I. C. Henderson and E. Frei III, *Cancer Treat. Rep.* 63(1-12): 1927-1952 (1979).
42. J. Liesmonn, R. J. Bett, C. D. Heas, and B. Hoogstralen, *Cancer Treat. Rep.* 65(9-10): 883-885 (1981).
43. S. M. Kupchan and R. M. Schubert, *Science* 185: 791 (1974).
44. *Compilation of the National Chinese Herbs.* The People's Publisher, Beijing, 1980.
45. K. I. Li, Y. L. Wang, C. P. Hsu, P. L. Chang, and W. Chao, *Yao Hsueh T'ung bao* 15(9): 43-45 (1980).
46. J. Arai, Y. Koyama, T. Suenaga and T. Morita, *J. Antibiotics, Ser. A* 16(3): 132-137 (1963).
47. E. Fujita, T. Fujita, H. Katayama, and M. Shibuya, *J. Chem. Soc. (C)* 1674-1679 (1970).
48. E. Fujita and M. Taoka, *Chem. Pharm. Bull.* 20(8): 1752-1754 (1972).
49. E. Fujita, M. Taoka, M. Shibuya and T. Fujita, *J. Chem. Soc. Perkin I.* 2277-2281 (1973).
50. E. Fujita, J. Nagao, K. Kaneko, S. Nakazawa, and H. Kuroda, *Chem. Pharm. Bull.* 24(9): 2118-2127 (1976).
51. E. Fujita, Y. Nagao, N. Node, K. Kaneko, I. Nakazawa, and H. Kuroda, *Experientia* 32: 203-208 (1976).
52. T. Fujita, T. Tchihara, Y. Takeda, Y. Takaishi, and T. Jingu,

C. A. 93: 26578q.

53. S. H. Doug, C. J. Hua, C. Z. Wen, T. Marunaka, Y. Minami, and T. Fujita, *Chem. Pharm. Bull.* 30(1): 341-433 (1982).
54. H. D. Sun, Z. W. Lin, Y. Minami, Y. Takeda, and T. Fujita, *Yakugaku Zasshi* 102(9): 887-890 (1982).
55. G. G. Li, Y. L. Wang, Z. P. Xu, P. L. Zhaug, and W. Zhao, *Yaoxue Xuebao* 16(9): 667-671 (1981).
56. J. Kubo, I. Miura, K. Nakanishi, T. Kamikawa, T. Isobe, and T. Kubota, *J. Chem. Soc., Chem. Commun.* 16: 555-556 (1977).
57. X. R. Wang, Z. Q. Wang, P. C. Shi, and B. G. Zhou, *Zhong C'aoyao* 13(6): 11-13 (1982).
58. I. Kubo, I. Miura, T. Kamikawa, T. Isobe, and T. Kubota, *Chem. Lett.* 11: 1289-1292 (1977).
59. M. Node, N. Ito, K. Fuji, and E. Fujita, *Chem. Pharm. Bull.* 30(7): 2639-2640 (1982).
60. E. Fujita, T. Fujita, and M. Shibuya, *Tetrahedron Letters* 27: 3153-3162 (1966).
61. G. K. Trivedi and I. Kubo, *J. Chromatography* 179: 219-221 (1979).
62. M. Taniguchi, M. Yamaguchi, I. Kubo, and T. Kubota, *Argric Biol. Chem.* 43(1): 71-74 (1979).
63. T. L. Wang, C. P. Chi, and K. H. Sheng, *Zhong C'aoyao* 12(1): 20-21 (1981).
64. Honan Institute of Medical Sciences, Honan Medical College, Yennan Institute of Botany, Cheng Chow Chemicopharmaceutical Plant. *K'ohsueh T'ungbao* 23: 53 (1978).
65. T. M. Chang, Z. Y. Chen, T. H. Chao, Q. Z. Zhao, H. D. Sun, and Z. W. Liu, *K'ohsueh T'ungbao* 25: 1051-1055 (1981).
66. E. Fujita, T. Fujita, and Y. Nagao, *Chem. Pharm. Bull.* 18(11): 2343-2345 (1971).
67. T. Fujita, I. Masuda, S. Takao, and E. Fujita, *J. Chem. Soc. Perkin I.* 19: 2098-2102 (1976).
68. Y. Nagao, E. Fujita, T. Kohno, and M. Yagi, *Chem. Pharm. Bull.* 29(11): 3202-3207 (1981).
69. E. Fujita, Y. Nagao, T. Kohno, M. Matsuda, and M. Ozaki, *Chem. Pharm. Bull.* 29(11): 3208-3218 (1981).

70. Y. Nagao, N. Ito, T. Kohno, H. Kuroda, and E. Fujita, *Chem. Pharm. Bull.* 30(2): 727-729 (1982).
71. *Zhong Yao Da Tsu Dien,* Shang Hai Science and Technology Publisher, (1977).
72. T. Fujita, *J. Chem. Soc., Chem. Commun.* 5: 205 (1980).
73. I. Kubo, M. J. Pettei, K. Hirotsu, H. Tsuji, and T. Kubota, *J. Am. Chem. Soc.* 100: 628-630 (1978).
74. P. B. Oetrichs, P. J. Vallely, J. K. Macleod, and I. A. S. Lewis, *J. Nat. Prod.* 43(3): 414-416 (1980).
75. I. Kubo, T. Kamikawa, and T. Kubota, *Tetrahedron Letters* 30: 615-622 (1974).
76. I. Kubo, N. A. Khatwa, T. Kubota, and T. Taniguchi, *J. Nat. Prod.* 44(5): 593-595 (1981).
77. I. H. Hall, R. Kaiai, R. Y. Wu, K. Tagahara, and K. H. Lee, *J. Pharm. Sci.* 71: 1263-1267 (1982).
78. S. M. Kupchan, Y. Shizuri, T. Murae, J. C. Sweeny, H. R. Haynes, M. S. Sheu, J. C. Barrick, R. F. Bryan, D. Helm, and K. K. Wu, *J. Am. Chem. Soc.* 98: 5719-5720 (1976).
79. K. Koike, C. Bevelle, S. K. Talapatra, G. A. Cordell, and N. R. Farnsworth, *Chem. Pharm. Bull.* 28: 401-405 (1980).
80. G. A. Cordell and N. R. Farnsworth, *Lloydia* 40: 1-44 (1977).
81. J. Konopa, A. Matuszkiewicz, M. Hrabowska, and K. Onoszka, *Arzneim Forsch.* 24: 1741-1743 (1974).
82. S. M. Kupchan, C. W. Sigel, L. J. Guttman, R. J. Restive, and R. F. Bryan, *J. Am. Chem. Soc.* 94: 1353-1354 (1972).
83. S. M. Kupchan and G. Tsou, *J. Org. Chem.* 38: 1055-1056 (1973).
84. S. M. Kupchan, G. Tsou, and C. W. Sigel, *J. Org. Chem.* 38: 1420-1421 (1973).
85. H. M. Deutsch and L. H. Zalkow, *J. Nat. Prod.* 45(4): 390-392 (1982).
86. K. A. Parker and J. R. Andrade, *J. Org. Chem.* 44: 3964 (1979).
87. M. Ogura, G. A. Cordell, and N. R. Farnsworth, *Lloydia* 39: 255 (1976).
88. G. R. Pettit, J. J. Einck, P. Brown, T. B. Harvey, III, R. H. Ode, and C. P. Pase, *J. Nat. Prod.* 43(5): 600-616 (1980).
89. F. Bohlman, K. H. Knoll, C. Zdero, P. K. Mahanta, M.

Grenz, A. Suwita, D. Ehlers, N. L. Van, W. R. Abraham,and A. A. Natu, *Phytochemistry* 16: 965 (1977).
90. H. M. Deutsch and L. H. Zalwow, *J. Nat. Prod.* 45(4): 390-392 (1982).
91. M. M. Rao and D. G. I. Kingston, *J. Nat. Prod.* 45(5): 600-604 (1982).
92. J. S. Driscoll, G. F. Hazard, Jr., H. B. Wood, Jr., and A. Doldin, *Cancer Chemoth. Rep.* 2,4(2): 1-21 (1974).
93. K. V. Rao, T. J. McBride and J. J. Oleson, *Cancer Res.* 28: 1952-1954 (1968).
94. U. Sankana, H. Otsuka, Y. Kataoka, Y. Litaka, A. Hoshi, and K. Kuretani, *Chem. Pharm. Bull.* 29: 116-122 (1981).
95. U. Sankaw, Y. Ebizuka, T. Miyazaki, Y. Isomura, H. Otsuka, S. Shibata, and M. Inomata, *Chem. Pharm. Bull.* 25(9): 2392-2395 (1977).
96. S. M. Kupchan, A. Karim, and C. Marchs, *J. Org. Chem.* 34: 3912-3918 (1969).
97. K. Mori and M. Matsui, *Tetrahedron Letters* 26: 3467-3473 (1970).
98. R. Zelnik, D. Lavie, E. C. Levy, A. H. J. Wang, and I. C. Paul, *Tetrahedron Letters* 33: 1457-1467 (1977).
99. B. Yang, M. Qian, and Z. Chen, *Yaoxue Xuebao* 16: 837-841 (1981).
100. E. Schwenk, *Arzneim. Forsch.* 12: 1145-1149 (1969).
101. P. Chang, K. H. Lee, T. Shingu, I. H. Hall, and H.C. Huang, *J. Nat. Prod.* 45(2): 206-210, (1982).
102. A. M. Arnold, *Cancer Chemoth. Pharmacol.* 3: 71-80 (1979).
103. M. Rozencweig, D. D. VonHoff, J. E. Henney, and F. M. Muggia, *Cancer* 40: 334-342 (1977).
104. D. Roberts, S. Hilliard, and C. Peck, *Cancer Res.* 40: 4225 (1980).
105. D. C. Ayres and C. K. Lim, *Cancer Chemoth. Pharmacol.* 7: 99 (1982).
106. J. D. Loike, *Cancer Chemoth. Pharmacol.* 7: 103 (1982).
107. J. C. Yalowich, D. W. Fry, and I. D. Goldman, *Cancer Research.* 42: 3648-3652 (1982).
108. R. E. Slayton, J. A. Blessing and G. Delgado, *Cancer Treat.*

Rep. 66(8): 1669-1671 (1982).

109. M. J. O'connell, J. Anderson, J. M. Merrill, J. M. Bennett, J. H. Glick, C. W. Bernard, R. S. Neiman, and H. S. Brodovsky, *Cancer Treat. Rep.* 66(12): 2021-2025 (1982).
110. B. F. Issell, C. Tihon, and M. E. Curvy, *Cancer Chemother. Pharmacol.* 7: 113 (1982).
111. W. J. Gensder, C. D. Murphy, and M. H. Trammell, *J. Med. Chem.* 20(5): 635-644 (1976).
112. M. C. Wani, H. L. Taylor, and M. E. Wall, *J. Am. Chem. Soc.* 93: 2325-2327 (1971).
113. E. Hamel, C. M. Lin, and D. G. Johns, *Cancer Treat. Rep.* 66(6): 1381-1386 (1982).
114. P. B. Schiff, J. Fant, and S. B. Horwitz, *Nature* 277: 665-667 (1979).
115. D. G. I. Kingston, D. R. Hawkins, and L. Ovington, *J. Nat. Prod.*, 45(4): 466-470 (1982).
116. J. Parness, D. G. I. Kingston, R. G. Powell, C. Harracksingh, and S. B. Horwitz, *Biochem. Biophys. Res. Comm.* 105: 1082-1089 (1982).
117. I. S. Johnson, J. G. Armstrong, M. Gorman, and J. P. Burnett, Jr., *Cancer Res.* 23: 1390-1427 (1963).
118. S. M. Sieber, J. A. R. Mead, and R. H. Adamson, *Cancer Treat. Rep.* 60(8): 1127-1139 (1976).
119. G. C. Told, W. J. Griffing, W. R. Gibson, and D. M. Morton, *Cancer Treat. Rep.* 63(1): 35-41 (1979).
120. D. V. Jackson, Jr., V. S. Setti, C. L. Spurr, and J. M. McWhorter, *Cancer Res.* 41: 1466-1469 (1981).
121. M. Valdivieso, A. Y. Bedikian, G. P. Bodey, and E. J. Freireich, *Cancer Treat. Rep.* 65: 877-879 (1981).
122. D. V. Jaskin, M. C. Castle, D. G. Poplack, and R. A. Bender, *Cancer Res.* 40: 722-724 (1980).
123. R. G. Powell, D. Weisleder, and C. R. Smith, *Tetrahedron Letters* 11: 815-818 (1970).
124. R. G. Powell, D. Weisleder, and C. R. Smith, Jr., *J. Pharm. Sci.* 61(8): 1227-1230 (1972).
125. C. R. Smith, Jr., R. G. Powell, and K. L. Mikolajzak, *Cancer Treat. Rep.* 60(8): 1157-1170 (1976).
126. G. E. Ma, L. T. Lin, T. Y. Chao, and H. C. Fan, *Huaxue*

Xuebao 35: 201-208 (1977).
127. G. E. Ma, C. N. Lu,and G. J. Fan, *Yaoxue Tongbao* 17(4): 205-206 (1982).
128. M. E. Wall, M. C. Mani, C. E. Cook, K. H. Palmer, and A. T. McPhall, *J. Am. Chem. Soc.* 88: 3888-3890 (1966).
129. G. H. Svoboda, G. A. Poore, P. J. Simpson, and G. B. Boder, *J. Pharm. Sci.* 55: 758-768 (1966).
130. G. H. Svoboda, M. J. Sweeney, and W. D. Walkling, *J. Pharm. Sci.* 60: 333 (1971).
131. K. V. Rao, R. Wilson, and B. Cummings, *J. Pharm. Sci.* 59: 1501-1502 (1970).
132. K. V. Rao, *J. Pharm. Sci.* 59: 1608-1611 (1970).
133. K. W. Kohn, M. J. Waring, D. G. Laubiger, and C. A. Friedman, *Cancer Research* 35: 71-76 (1975).
134. B. Salles, J. Y. Charcosset, and A. J. Sablon, *Cancer Treat. Rep.* 66(2): 327-338 (1982).
135. J. B. Lepcq, C. Gosse, N. D. Xuong, S. Cros, and C. Paoletti, *Cancer Res.* 36: 3067-3076 (1976).
136. P. Juret, J. F. Heron, J. E. Couette, T. Delozier, and J. Y. LeTalaer, *Cancer Treat. Rep.* 66(11): 1909-1916 (1982).
137. Z. X. Huang and Z. H. Li, *Huaxue Xue-bao* 38: 535-542 (1980).
138. M. H. Wang, *Yaoxue Tongbao* 38: 535-542 (1981).
139. M. L. Sethi, *J. Nat. Prod.* 42: 187-196 (1979).
140. K. Y. Robet, Z. Cheng, S. J. Yan, and C. C. Cheng, *J. Med. Chem.* 21: 199-203 (1978).
141. F. R. Stermitz, J. P. Gillespie, L. G. Amoros, R. Romero, and T. A. Stermitz, *J. Med. Chem.* 18: 708-713 (1975).
142. G. A. Cordell and N. R. Farnsworth, *Lloydia* 40: 17-19 (1977).
143. C. C. J. Culvenor, *J. Pharm. Sci.* 57: 1112 (1968).
144. M. Kugelman, W. Chin, M. Axelrod, T. J. McBride, and K. V. Rao, *Lloydia* 39: 125 (1976).
145. D. S. Poster, S. Bruno, J. Penta, and J. S. MacDonald, *Cancer Treat. Rep.* 65: 53-55 (1981).
146. G. Powls, M. M. Ames, and J. S. Kovach, *Cancer Research* 39: 3564-3570 (1979).
147. J. A. Edgar, L. W. Smith, and C. C. J. Culvenor, *Mol. Pharm.*

6: 402-406 (1970).

148. I. C. Hsu, K. A. Robertson, R. C. Shumaker, and J. R. Allen, *Re. Commu. Chem. Pathol. Pharmacol.* 11: 99-106 (1975).

149. K. A. Robertson, *Cancer Research* 42: 8-13 (1982).

150. J. R. Allen, I. C. Hsu, and L. A. Carstens, *Cancer Research* 35: 997-1002 (1975).

151. R. Schoental, *Cancer Research* 35: 2020-2023 (1975).

152. S. M. Kupchan, A. T. Sneden, A. R. Branfman, G. A. Howie, L. J. Rebhum, W. E. McIvor, R. W. Wang, and T. C. Schnaitman, *J. Med. Chem.* 21: 31-37 (1978).

153. A. P. Chahinian, C. Nogeire, T. Ohnuma, M. L. Greenberg, M. Sivak, I. S. Jaffrey, and J. F. Holland, *Cancer Treat. Rep.* 63: 1953-1960 (1979).

154. B. A. Chabner, A. S. Levine, B. L. Johnson, and R. C. Young, *Cancer Treat. Rep.* 62: 429-433 (1978).

155. I. S. Jaffrey and J. M. Denefrio, *Cancer Treat. Rep.* 64: 193-194 (1980).

156. R. F. Luduena and M. C. Roach, *Biochemistry* 20(15): 4444-4450 (1981).

157. R. T. Eagan, E. T. Creager, J. N. Ingle, S. Frytak, and J. Rubin, *Cancer Treat. Rep.* 62: 1577-1579 (1978).

158. M. J. O'connell, A. Shni, J. Rubin, and C. G. Moertel, *Cancer Treat. Rep.* 62: 1237-1238 (1978).

159. H. M. Pinedo, *Cancer Chemotherapy, Annual 3,* Elsevler. New York, 142-143, 1981.

160. A. T. Sneden and G. L. Beemsterbeer, *J. Nat. Prod.* 43: 637-640 (1980).

161. A. T. Sneden, W. C. Sumner, Jr., and S. M. Kupchan, *J. Nat. Prod.* 45(5): 624-628 (1982).

162. A. O. Ajibola, *J. Nat. Prod.* 43(4): 482-486 (1980).

163. S. M. Kupchan, R. J. Hemingway, J. R. Knox, S. J. Barboutis, D. Werner, and M. A. Barboutis, *J. Pharm. Sci.* 56: 603-608 (1967).

164. E. R. Bianchi and J. R. Cole, *J. Pharm. Sci.* 58: 589-591 (1969).

165. K. Y. Robet, Z. Cheng, S. J. Yan, and C. C. Cheng, *J. Med. Chem.* 21(2): 199-203 (1978).

166. H. Y. Hsu, Y. P. Chen, and M. Hong, *The Chemical Constituents of Oriental Herbs,* Oriental Healing Arts Institute, 1982.
167. C. S. Lin, *The Chemistry of Constituents of Chinese Herbs,* Science Publishing House, 1977.
168. P. G. Sarath, S. P. Gunasekera, G. A. Cordell, and N. R. Farnsworth, *Phytochemistry* 19(6): 1213-1218 (1980).
169. S. D. Jolad, J. J. Hoffmann, J. R. Cole, M. S. Fempesta, and R. B. Bates, *J. Org. Chem.* 46(9): 1946-1947 (1981).
170. K. Hayashi, K. Wada, H. Mitsuhashi, and H. Bando, *Chem. Pharm. Bull.* 28(6): 1954-1958 (1980).
171. P. M. Dewick and D. E. Jackson, *Phytochemistry* 20: 2277-2280 (1981).
172. M. V. Nadkarni, P. B. Maury, and J. L. Hartwell, *J. Am. Chem. Soc.* 74: 280-281 (1952); 75: 1308-1312 (1953).
173. H. Limburg et al., *Planta Medica* 22: 348-357 (1972).
174. K. Sheth, E. Bianchi, R. Wiedhope, and J. R.Cole, *J. Pharm. Sci.* 62: 139-140 (1973).
175. A. A. Saleh et al. *J. C. S. Perkin I.* 5: 1090-1097 (1980).
176. D. G. I. Kingston and M. M. Rao, *Planta Medica* 39(3): 230 (1980).
177. T. T. Oleson, *C. A.* 68: 28403m (1968).
178. E. R. Trumbull and R. J. Cole, *J. Pharm. Sci.* 58: 176-178 (1969); J. R. Cole, E. Bianchi, and E. R.Trumbull, *J. Pharm. Sci.* 58: 175-176 (1969).
179. H. S. Dan, *Yaoxue Xuebao* 16(2): 155 (1981).
180. C. C. Lin, J. M. Ma, and J. Lin, *Beijingdaxue Xuebao, Ziran Kexneban* 127: 94-96 (1981).
181. S. M. Kupchan, Y. Aynenchi, J. M. Cassady, H. K. Sohnoes, and A. L. Burlingame, *J. Org. Chem.* 34: 3867-3875 (1969).
182. S. M. Kupchan, J. C. Hemingway, J. M. Cassady, J. R. Knox, A. T. McPhail, and G. A. Sim, *J. Am. Chem. Soc.* 89: 465-466 (1967).
183. S. M. Kupchan, J. E. Kelsey, M. Maruyama, J. M. Cassady, J. C. Hemingway, and J. R. Knox, *J. Org. Chem.* 34: 3876-3883 (1969).
184. S. M. Kupchan, J. M. Cassady, J. Bailey, and J. R. Knox, *J. Pharm. Sci.* 54: 1703-1704 (1965).

185. A. Ulubelen, M. E. Caldwell, and J. R. Cole, *J. Pharm. Sci.* 54: 1214-1216 (1965).
186. S. M. Kupchan, M. A. Eakin, and A. M. Thomas, *J. Med. Chem.* 14: 1147-1152 (1971).
187. P. B. Oelrichs, P. J. Vallely, J. K. Macleod, and I. A. S. Levis, *J. Nat. Prod.* 43(3): 414-416 (1980).
188. A. G. Gonzales, V. Darias, G. Alonsa, and E. Esterez, *Planta Medica* 40(2): 179-184 (1980).
189. S. Nagumo, K. Izawa, K. Higashiyama, and M. Nagai, *Yakugaku Zasshi* 100(4): 427-433 (1980).
190. D. A. Gairnes, O. Ekundayo, and D. G. I. Kingston, *J. Nat. Prod.* 43(4): 495-497 (1980).
191. S. M. Kupchan, R. J. Hemingway, P. Coggen, A. T. McPhail, and G. A. Sim, *J. Am. Chem. Soc.* 90: 2982 (1968).
192. S. M. Kupchan, C. W. Sigel, M. J. Matz, J. A. Saenzrena, R. C. Haltiwanger, and R. S. Bryan, *J. Am. Chem. Soc.* 92: 4476-4477 (1970).
193. R. P. Rorris, G. A. Cordell, and N. R. Farnsworth, *J. Nat. Prod.* 43(5): 641-643 (1980).
194. J. Y. Lin, K. Y. Tserug, L. T. Lin, and T. C. Tung, *Nature* 227: 292-294 (1970).
195. T. Utika and A. Tanimura, *Chem. Pharm. Bull.* 9: 43-53 (1961).
196. U. C. Bhargava and B. A. Westfall, *J. Pharm. Sci.* 57: 1674-1677 (1968).
197. R. Kasai, T. Shingu, R. Y. Wu, I. H. Hall, and K. H. Lee, *J. Nat. Prod.* 45(3): 317-320 (1982).
198. O. M. Parkash, D. S. Bhakuri, and R. S. Kapil, *J. Chem. Soc., Perkin I.* 5: 1305-1308 (1979).
199. P. W. L. Quesne, J. E. Larrahondo, and R. F. Raffauf, *J. Nat. Prod.* 43(3): 353-359 (1980).
200. R. Kojima, S. Fukushima, A. Ueno, and Y. Saiki, *Chem. Pharm. Bull.* 18: 2555-2563 (1970).
201. R. G. Powell and C. R. Smith, Jr., *J. Nat. Prod.* 44(1): 86-90 (1981).
202. H. Lessner, U. Jonson, V. Loeb, and W. Larsen, *Cancer Chemother. Rep.* 27: 33-44 (1963).
203. D. C. Stolinsky, E. M. Jacobs, J. R. Bateman, and J. L.

Hazen, *Cancer Chemother. Rep.* 51: 25-34 (1967).

204. P. R. Ravikumor, P. Hammesfahr, and C. J. Sin, *J. Pharm. Sci.* 68(7): 900-903 (1979).
205. J. Nienhaus, M. Stoll, and F. Vester, *Experientia* 26: 523-526 (1970).
206. S. M. Kupchan, N. Yokoyama, and B. S. Thyagarajan, *J. Pharm Sci.* 50: 164-167 (1961).
207. A. Ulubelen, M. E. Caldwell, and J. R. Cole, *J. Pharm. Sci.* 54: 1214-1216 (1965).
208. A. Ulubelen and J. R. Cole, *J. Pharm. Sci.* 55: 1368-1370 (1968).
209. M. E. Wall, M. C. Wani, C. E. Cook, K. H. Palmer, A. T. McPhail, and G. A. Sim, *J. Am. Chem. Soc.* 88: 3888-3890 (1966).
210. C. G. Moertel, *Cancer Chemother. Rep., Part 1* 56: 95 (1972).
211. S. M. Kupchan and A. Karim, *Lloydia* 39: 223 (1976).
212. The Chinese Medicinal Institute, Chinese Traditional Medicine Academy, *Xin Yiyao Zazhi* 2: 9; 3: 51 (1979).
213. T. Miyazaki and M. Nishijima, *Chem. Pharm. Bull.* 29: 3611-3616 (1981).
214. G. Chihara, Y. Maeda, N. Hamura, Y. Arai, and F. Fukuoka, *Nature* 225: 943-944 (1970).
215. G. Chihara, J. Hamuro, Y. Maeda, T. Sasaki, and F. Fukuoka, *Nature* 222: 687-688 (1970).
216. G. Chihara, J. Hamuro, Y. Maeda, Y. Arai, and F. Fukuoka, *Cancer Res.* 30: 2776-2781 (1970).
217. S. M. Kupchan, K. K. Chakravarti, and N. Yakoyama, *J. Pharm. Sci.* 52: 985-988 (1963).
218. Y. Nishihama, K. Masuda, M. Yamaki, S. Takagi, and K. Sakina, *Planta Medica* 43: 28-33 (1981).
219. S. Takagi, M. Yamaki, K. Mashihama, and K. Sakina, *Yakugaku Zasshi* 101: 657-659 (1981).
220. K. Koike, G. A. Cordell, N. R. Farnsworth, A. A. Freer, C. J. Gilmore, and G. A. Sim, *Tetrahedron Letters,* 36(9): 1167-1172 (1980).
221. F. Panthiere and C. A. Coltman, Jr., *Cancer* 27: 835-841 (1971).

222. W. R. Jondorf, B. J. Abbott, N. H. Greenberg, and J. A. R. Mead, *Chemotherapy* 16: 109-129 (1971).
223. Z. D. Wu, L. X. Li, S. N. Su, L. M. Zerg, and K. H. Long. *Zhongshan Xuebao, Ziran Kexueban* 2: 113-115 (1981).
224. M. D. Antoun, D. Abramson, R. L. Tyson, C. J. Chang, J. L. McLaughlin, G. Peck, and J. M. Cassady, *J. Nat. Prod.* 44(5): 579-585 (1981).
225. S. M. Kupchan, S. J. Barboutis, J. R. Knox, and C. A. L. Cam, *Science* 150: 1827-1828 (1965).
226. S. M. Kupchan, A. P. Davies, S. J. Barboutis, H. K. Schnoes, and A. L. Burlingame, *J. Am. Chem. Soc.* 89: 5718-5719 (1967).
227. M. C. Wani, H. L. Taylor, M. E. Wall, P. Coggon, and A. T. McPhail, *J. Am. Chem. Soc.* 93: 2325-2326 (1971).
228. R. L. Hanson, H. A. Lardy, and S. M. Kupchan, *Science* 168: 378-380 (1970).
229. J. A. Hembree, C. J. Chang, J. L. McLaughlin, and J. M. Cassady, *Phytochemistry* 18(10): 1691-1694 (1979).
230. J. A. Hembree, C. J. Chang, J. L. McLaughlin, and J. M. Cassady, *Experientia* 36(1): 28-29 (1980).
231. I. H. Hall, K. Tagahara, and K. H. Lee, *J. Pharm. Sci.* 71: 741-744 (1982).
232. Y. F. Liou, I. H. Hall, and K. H. Lee, *J. Pharm. Sci.* 71: 745-749 (1982).
233. A. Kato, Y. Hashimoto, and M. Kidokoro, *J. Nat. Prod.* 42(2): 159-162 (1979).
234. K. H. Lee, K. Tayohara, H. Suzuki, R. Y. Yu, M. Haruna, and I. H. Hall, *J. Nat. Prod.* 44(5): 530-535 (1981).
235. C. Bounthanh, C. Bergmann, J. P. Beck, M. M. Berrurier, and R. Anton, *Planta Medica* 41(1): 21-28 (1981).
236. *Zhong C'aoyao Hsueh,* Ian-su People's Publishers, (1979).

Index

B

C

D

E

F

G

H

I

M

N

O

P

Q

R

S

T

U

V

W

X

Z

Structure-Activity Relationship Analysis of Chinese Anticancer Drugs and Related Plants

- ***Surveys over 120 species of plants, many of them used in Chinese traditional or folk medicine to treat cancer***
- ***Reports on the scientific screening of compounds isolated from plants that have shown cytotoxic and/or antitumor activity***
- ***Examines the structures of active compounds and mechanisms of action for sesquiterpenes, diterpenes, triterpenes, steroids, alkaloids, and others***
